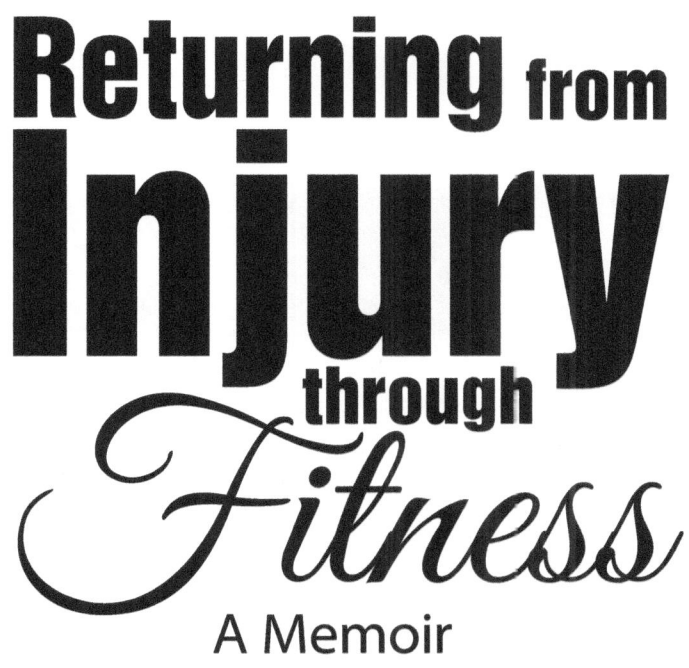

Returning from Injury through Fitness

A Memoir

Robert G. Beauchamp, PhD

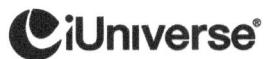

RETURNING FROM INJURY THROUGH FITNESS
A MEMOIR

iUniverse books may be ordered through booksellers or by contacting:

iUniverse
1663 Liberty Drive
Bloomington, IN 47403
www.iuniverse.com
1-800-Authors (1-800-288-4677)

Because of the dynamic nature of the Internet, any web addresses or links contained in this book may have changed since publication and may no longer be valid. The views expressed in this work are solely those of the author and do not necessarily reflect the views of the publisher, and the publisher hereby disclaims any responsibility for them.

Any people depicted in stock imagery provided by Thinkstock are models, and such images are being used for illustrative purposes only. Certain stock imagery © Thinkstock.

ISBN: 978-1-5320-1778-0 (sc)
ISBN: 978-1-5320-1777-3 (e)

Library of Congress Control Number: 2017937160

Print information available on the last page.

iUniverse rev. date: 08/29/2017

Acknowledgement

Thanks to my family for all their caring and support.

Contents

Introduction

I became a senior person in February 2016. While this was traumatic, I am physically and mentally active and feel quite good. With the exception of nearly six months in 2015, I was exercising regularly for nearly thirty-five years. During which, the quality of my life steadily improved and I owe this to becoming and remaining fit.

In May 2015, I fell on the deck of my getaway house in West Virginia and tore the ligament in my right knee that controls motion. This accident resulted in having to undergo knee surgery, followed by periods of convalescing, recovery, and extensive rehabilitation to regain my abilities I subsequently lost. I also describe injuries that occurred earlier in my life that required periods of rehabilitation and the determination that would return me to normalcy. These earlier accidents made me understand the importance of undertaking a program of regular and vigorous exercise to maintain a healthy existence. This book also includes experiences while exercising and how they have enhanced my life.

The story I wish to share is not unique to me alone. There are many senior or nearly senior-aged individuals who had similar experiences that motivated them to participate in exercise programs. While motives and experiences associated with exercising can be similar, we have much to learn from the feelings and insights that are evoked while undertaking this commitment.

There are several reasons why I wish to share about being active and regaining fitness following an accident. First, I am acutely aware that through sharing, I'm able to see how important exercise has been in aiding me deal with the kinds of crises we all have to contend with in our lives. These include illness, injuries, relocating, divorce, others. As a result of exercising regularly, I've been rewarded by not only increases in strength, overall good health, and endurance but an increase in my inner strength as well. Second, this book may serve to motivate others to exercise, especially those who feel it's beyond their ability—that they're too old or too out of shape to have any chance of becoming fit. In addition, some may have concluded that as a result of illness or disability, they wouldn't be able to endure the physical demands or discomfort that can accompany an exercise program.

I strongly contend that exercise not only improves the quality of our lives, including our physical, emotional, and intellectual abilities, but also helps us to fully appreciate our spirituality. As we progress in achieving fitness and improving our health, we may also discover the desire to explore the depth and meaning of our lives. Exercise demands concentration and dedication. Attaining spiritual fulfillment also requires concentration and dedication. Exercising may encourage us to participate more fully in mental and spiritual activities and ultimately reap the benefits. This is a lifelong commitment. There are no quick or easy fixes and I'm convinced the benefits far outweigh the costs.

This book covers a period from my childhood, through teenage years, early adulthood and finally maturity. The emphasis is on events and experiences that required me to make life sustaining decisions and develop pathways to heal and enrich my life.

Along with reading this book and receiving professional guidance, others may gain insight into the importance of being healthy and fit. With the support of family and friends, along with commitment, we can become and remain rejuvenated. Even more importantly, this resolve can prepare us to deal effectively with the challenges of everyday living. It can be a fulfilling and exhilarating experience, as it has been and continues to be for me.

2

$\mathcal{E}$arly On

To begin, I wish to identify various experiences that eventually led me to consider becoming healthy. I provide background information about where I grew up, influences that both plagued and motivated me, and why I eventually decided to become both educated and healthy.

Having moved from Holyoke, Massachusetts to Staten Island, New York at the age of twelve, I found myself in a very different environment. Staten Island was not as sparsely populated as in and around Holyoke. Living there as a child and pre-teen, I was able to play and explore the surrounding forest and parks with my dog and friends. In the winter, portions of the parks would be flooded with water, so when ice would form, I would enjoy ice-skating, especially with my mother since she was good. Staten Island didn't offer that opportunity. As in most urban areas, there were parks, but they weren't easily accessible from where I lived and didn't have any winter ice on which to skate.

The Island, as fondly referred to by its residents, is located in New York Bay between New Jersey and Brooklyn. It can be reached by two bridges extending from New Jersey and also includes the Verrazano Bridge that connects the Island with Brooklyn. In addition, there are ferryboats that travel across the bay between the Island and Manhattan. Even though it's close to New Jersey, it remains part of New York as one of the five boroughs. Ferryboats travel between it and Manhattan and the views surrounding the Bay are fabulous. Even though the Island is relatively near other highly populated boroughs, it has numerous parks with small lakes and is not as congested as the others.

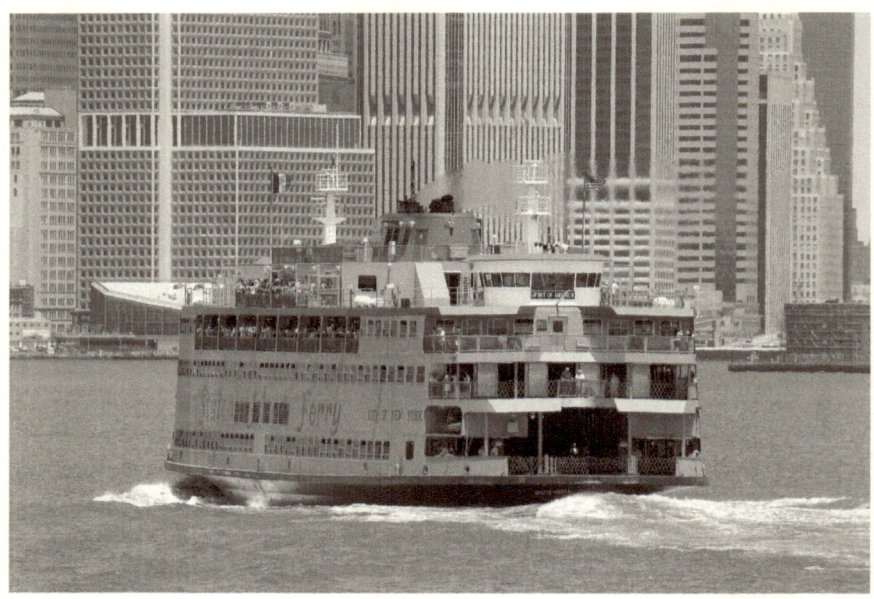

The ferryboat ride is a popular tourist attraction for those visiting New York. It provides excellent views of the Statue of Liberty, Governor's Island, and the Manhattan skyline that consists of nearly cloud-touching skyscrapers. While the Twin Towers are no longer there, a new building complex has been built in the same location. I haven't seen this complex, but when I do I will likely feel deep sadness over the loss of the Towers and many of its occupants.

The ferry's main mission is to transport commuters to Manhattan in the morning so they can make their way to work and bring them back in the evening. It also transports other passengers and cars traveling in or out of the area, as well as those interested in viewing the Statue of Liberty and the Manhattan skyline. When the ferry docks, commuters typically race off the boat with a single purpose; rushing from the terminal to disappear into dark cavities in the streets making their way downward to subways that carry them to their destination.

As a teenager, I would normally sit inside the main cabin of a ferry as opposed to standing outside near the railings. Unfortunately, it wouldn't be long before the cabin would be filled with cumulus-like clouds of tobacco smoke from every conceivable source such as cigars, pipes, and cigarettes. They all contributed to this haze and it appeared that everyone smoked something. It wouldn't be long before I found myself nearly suffocating and would bolt outside onto the deck to breathe fresh air.

My parents were in the midst of divorcing, and it was decided that I would live with my mother. She wanted to be near her family, who lived on the Island. My father was going to live and work in Manhattan. It was clear he didn't want me with him as a full-time responsibility. I felt abandoned and also angry. To hurt him, I falsely told him I would rather be with my mother. Even though we weren't very close and he occasionally frightened me with his gruffness and demanding demeanor, I looked up to him and felt protected when he was near. He was also respected by the way others treated him and how they treated me. My father was the type of person who seemingly filled a large space when he was near, but when he wasn't, it seemed he had vanished forever. Except for my mother, there was no one available to look up to or feel protected and I felt vulnerable.

I enrolled in eighth grade at a public school and my mother rented a small apartment nearby. At first, making friends was difficult, but soon I found suitable companions. After completing elementary school, I enrolled in a religion-oriented junior high school. My mother felt I needed male guidance, and she thought the teachers would provide it. This never proved well founded. I found the teachers frightening by the way they scolded students. Occasionally, they would threaten to strike a student with an open hand or even a fist. Even though this might have been acceptable practice, it was terrifying to witness. I recall how a teacher would frequently glare at students in class for some unknown reason. Unfortunately, I sat directly in front of him and any moment expected to be scolded. While this didn't occur, anticipating such aggression was nearly experiencing the event. I wasn't able to last beyond the first year. I felt this was not the environment where I could learn, so I convinced my mother to enroll me in a local public high school. In addition, a teacher whom I respected had resigned from the school and accepted a position at this high school.

I soon discovered this school had the qualities I longed for, including sports, friendly teachers, and also girls — so many I could hardly believe it. At first, I felt awkward around them but soon realized they were attracted to me. Some girls would wait outside my classroom and walk with me to my next class. Even though I was shy, I soon gained confidence and began to easily circulate among them and eventually dated several.

My fear of teachers quickly disappeared. They were not inclined to scold or intimidate students and appeared to be in control of their behavior. They were helpful and not threatening. Drinking on school property was naturally not permitted, however, smoking by students was common. They would find places within the school grounds to smoke a cigarette.

I quickly made friends and eventually played varsity football—a sport that bestowed on me considerable stature. Making friends was easy since being on the team gave me lots of exposure and importance. I was invited to parties and many students wanted to be my friend. It was an uplifting experience to be popular. My situation of being from a broken family was not unique, and playing football helped me to deal with this circumstance. Those who eventually became my friend had similar family situations, such as having a single parent, apartment living, and very little money.

To conserve money and be close to school, we moved from an area of primarily private homes to a community of low- to middle-class apartments with a few private homes. The homes and apartments appeared older than where we previously lived. The apartment we rented was near the ferryboat terminal, where those traveling to and from Manhattan made their landing. Since it only cost five cents, occasionally I would take the ferry to gaze out across the bay and wonder what happened in my life that brought me here. Gone was the rolling countryside surrounding Holyoke, my boyhood friends and the places I roamed and explored and the days when I hiked the Berkshire hills with my dog and even my mother. I often felt depressed as I realized I likely would not have that secure and protected life again.

As a teenager, I was introduced to smoking and drinking. Since most of my newly acquired friends were older, they often smoked and drank beer. If I was going to get along and be accepted, I was going to have to do what they did. At sixteen, I was tall for my age and therefore able to pass for the legal age of eighteen to be served some form of alcohol. Most of the time I could buy beer from liquor stores without being asked for proof of age. At the time, drinking two or three beers was sufficient to make me feel dizzy and disoriented.

One evening a friend and I decided we would drink an entire case of beer we purchased earlier and stashed away for just the right time. We must have been insane to think we could drink that much beer. That suggests how overly optimistic teenagers can be. Hoisting the case of beer on my shoulders, we went to a nearby deserted field and began opening the beer cans and draining them as fast as we could. It wasn't very long when less than two six packs were consumed. Both of us couldn't stand up any longer, and our speech was so slurred we couldn't understand what the other was saying. Feelings of dizziness and weightlessness soon gave way to waves of nausea. We finally felt relief following our chorus of retching that broke the stillness of evening. I was amazed that no one heard and came to see what was happening. It was quite a while before we recovered from that episode. Although it didn't cure us; it only made us realize what would happen if we weren't careful about how much we drank. We continued to drink, but much less and at a slower pace and discovered we could drink more if we just cut down on the rate of consumption. As I reflect, it's difficult to understand why it took so long to come to that conclusion. Although at that age, arriving at some conclusions is not always rapid or reliable.

As a teenager, I was free to roam the streets either alone or with friends. My mother didn't have the time or energy to control my behavior. She felt alone and burdened with sole responsibility of raising me. Occasionally she depended on alcohol to help her cope with anxiety and despair. Since I didn't wish to witness this, I often walked the streets at night and developed a sense of self-confidence that I could take care of myself no matter what I might confront. I didn't fear being out alone, even though some streets were filthy with litter and inhabited by vagrants searching for money to buy liquor. Some began to see me as one who had no more than they possessed and likely felt I was poor; and poor we were!

The first apartment we lived in didn't have a refrigerator, and we had to share the bathroom with another family. In the summer, we would put our food in a neighbor's refrigerator or place it outside on window sills or on the porch. Money was scarce. My father would send money, especially when I would call and asked him. At first, my mother didn't work until she was hired as a clerk in a dry-cleaning establishment—a job she would hold for nearly seven years until she remarried.

Smoking was a prerequisite for being accepted by my peers, and I didn't find this difficult since most of my heroes on the screen, such as Humphrey Bogart and John Wayne, often smoked. When smoking a cigarette while acting out their roles, it added additional dimensions to their characters, such as controlled strength and wisdom—behavioral traits I both lacked and coveted. I recall John Wayne in the role of a marine corps sergeant in a popular action movie offering a cigarette to a distraught marine officer to calm him down after surviving a beach landing. This linkage of cigarettes while dealing with a very stressful moment impressed me, especially since it was promoted by one of my favorite actors.

Smoking a cigarette also contributed to making a person appear more attractive, rugged looking, and even respected—attributes I wished were part of my identity. In his roles, Humphrey Bogart always appeared very masculine and in control of any situation when there was a cigarette between his lips. This type of behavior personified toughness or callousness, which I perceived to be impenetrable by any evil force. For me, smoking even demonstrated manhood and strength. At that time in my life, I valued these traits since I wasn't sure of who I was and I possessed precious little self-confidence. Therefore, I vainly attempted to mimic the personalities of my heroes on the screen and tried to integrate them into my own behavior. Smoking was an important vehicle for attempting this transformation.

At the time, cigarette ads and commercials demonstrated how wonderful it was to smoke. On billboards, the radio, and especially television ads were constantly reminding me how incredibly cool it was. There was no way to escape this barrage of advertisements. In my mind, anyone who was important smoked. Both my parents, as well as most of my relatives smoked over the course of their lives and may have been the demise of many of them.

As I grew into manhood, smoking continued to be a part of my life. When I was an adolescent, my parents, especially my mother, tried to make it clear they didn't want me to smoke even though their own cigarette smoke permeated the surrounding air. I once felt honored by my father when he permitted me to keep a lit cigarette in my hand so I could set off fireworks on the Fourth of July. I felt he was treating me like an adult. Since It was expected that men smoked, it heralded the arrival of manhood. Smoking was so pervasive when I was a teenager that one of my relatives suggested I should smoke a cigarette after finishing a meal since it would help digest the food. As I continued smoking, it was not very long before the desire to have a cigarette became overwhelming. This linkage of smoking to eating strengthened over the years.

Smoking and drinking alcohol were strongly linked together. I soon discovered they complemented each other both in images and taste. Any manner of drink appeared to taste much better while smoking a cigarette. Additionally, most anyone appeared sophisticated when smoking. It also seemed to provide an opportunity to be friendly toward the opposite sex by offering them a cigarette, lighting it, and sharing the pleasure of satisfying an addictive craving. My vision of a life that projected masculinity, attractiveness, excitement, and even intrigue was connected with both smoking cigarettes and drinking. I wasn't totally aware of it, but I was addicted to nicotine. I was also becoming dependent on alcohol and it reinforced my desire to smoke.

As I grew older, smoking became my everyday thing. It wasn't long before I was a pack-a-day smoker; smoking nearly two packs a day soon became common. My addiction became so extreme that when I ran out of cigarettes, I would scavenge butts off the ground or out of ashtrays to smoke what remained. When I was desperate for a cigarette, no butt was too far gone for me. There were instances when I even tried smoking the filter of a cigarette.

Smoking a cigarette precipitated an event that resulted in me wrecking my car the first time I drove it. As I was driving to attend a class at a local university, I dropped the cigarette I was smoking onto the car floor. As I reached down to retrieve it, my eyes left the road, and I inadvertently drove into a parked car. I demolished the front end of my car but hardly left a scratch on the other car. My car was no longer usable, and I had to get rid of it.

The adult world was a smoking world when I entered it in the 1950s. Most my friends and coworkers smoked. Even though I burned through many a shirt, tie, and even a pair of pants, I continued to smoke. I had to have a cigarette following a meal or when I drank any kind of liquid, especially beer. I smoked while I worked, when I would read, talk, and walk, and even just before I went to bed. If I woke up in the middle of the night, I would occasionally light up. When any kind of stress or anxiety crept into my life, I immediately reached for a cigarette. Essentially, most of my waking hours were spent smoking. In time, I developed a persistent cough and would find myself seriously out of breath when I hurried along at a brisk pace. Others told me that my clothes, furniture, blankets, rugs, curtains, the interior of my car, my body, and my hair smelled of tobacco smoke. There was no way I could escape its insults.

During the years prior to 1980, a healthy existence was not my bent even though there were brief periods when I would jog in neighborhoods where I lived or played tennis—an activity I thoroughly enjoyed but never became competent. Drinking, smoking cigarettes or even a cigar were my principal choices of recreation. The quality of my life continued to degenerate, and my ability to sustain some semblance of a fulfilling and responsible life was severely impaired. I managed to hold onto a reasonably good job. but my daily existence had become a series of activities in search of pleasure without any obvious purpose. I inherently knew that my survival was in jeopardy, although I was unmotivated and had no inclination to do much about it. I felt alone, confused, and without any clear vision of the future. Values such as a job, family, and friends, which at one point in my life were important, were not fully realized. I even doubted they ever had any importance. A failed marriage and neglected children left me with enormous guilt that further propelled me in search of self-gratification and avoid serious soul searching about what was important and where I was heading in life.

One evening I attended a party where everyone was drinking liquor. I decided to join in and soon I became incoherent. At one point when I was laughing, I struck my forehead on the edge of a chair. This resulted in injuring my eye and required medical attention. I immediately left the party and drove to the nearest hospital with the use of only one eye. Soon after I arrived, I was taken into the emergency room, and the doctor asked me what happened. When I explained the reason for the injury, he was surprised I had allowed myself to become so out of control. His reaction was a major blow to how I felt about myself. I began to realize I needed to make a major adjustment in my life and never again indulge in the use of alcohol that led to my loss of self-control. This realization became a major turning point in my life.

3

Change in Direction

In January 1955, while living in Maryland, I made several decisions that would have an impact on the directions I would take in my life. Since I was at the age where men were being drafted into the Army, I began thinking about enlisting in the U.S. Marine Corps Reserves. I would be able to satisfy my requirement of serving in the military and still attend college. I asked a friend his opinion of the reserves since he had joined a year earlier. His response was very positive, and he encouraged me to join. At the time, I was anticipating being drafted into the army to serve out my military requirement. Therefore, while attending college, I joined the reserves. This would allow me to remain in school while I served in the military. Being in the reserves was a very positive experience. The Marine Corps is a highly respected service with a stellar reputation. The time I spent as a marine taught me a great deal about myself, as well as this country. I'm sure any of our military services would do the same for its enlistees. The corps, as it's fondly referred to by its members, has a rich and coveted history. For example, it's the oldest military service in the United States. The reason the United States emblem is not part of the uniform is because the corps was created prior to the creation of the United States. This actually occurred in 1864 at a bar in Philadelphia, one year prior to the creation of the United States. Marines enjoy telling others how appropriate it was for the corps to be created in a bar knowing how much marines enjoy drinking.

My military service began on the day of my birthday, February 22, and I received an Honorable Discharge ten years later on February 22. My enlistment was initially for eight years and required four years of active duty and four years of serving in the reserves. After completing the required eight years of service, I reenlisted for two more years. The time spent in the corps taught me a great deal about its motto: duty, honor, and country. It may be difficult for others to understand the commitment and feelings associated with this motto. I was fortunate to have served in both the infantry and the air wing and developed a sense of pride about their missions. Additionally, keeping physically fit was important to perform all the rigorous activities marines are subjected to in training.

While serving in the reserves, I received a notice from the US Selective Service's draft office to report to the office in New York to receive a physical examination for induction into the US Army. This was very strange since I was already in the reserves. In attempting to contact the draft office and notify them about this error, I was informed that I needed to report for the physical exam or I would be arrested and forced to comply with the induction notice. I gathered all the papers associated with being in the reserves and arrived at the draft office. When I attempted to explain my situation to those in charge, they paid little attention and just ordered me to follow the others to the location for testing my literacy, followed by a physical exam. I felt I should comply with their directions and hopefully would find someone who would listen to my explanation about already being in the military. After I received a physical examination and took a written test, I finally was interviewed by an official. It was then I had the opportunity to explain that I was in the active Marine Corps reserves and didn't feel I was required to undergo this examination for induction into the army. When I presented the papers showing that I was a reservist, I received an apology and was informed they had no record of my enlistment. After my personnel record was updated, I was permitted to leave. It clearly impressed me that there can be occasions where an explanation of who one is may not be sufficient without proper documentation.

I felt privileged to serve in the Marine Corps with men who came from various walks of life. There were men with senior ranks who had served in WWII and Korea. There were high school graduates, college students and even those with PhD's in various disciplines. I became friends with a marine who earned a PhD in electrical engineering. I admired his intelligence, and it wasn't long before our conversations led me to seriously think about attending college. It was always in my mind to do so, but he made me realize how important it was to follow that path. I just needed to identify a subject to major in!

I had an important, if not a life changing experience when I was on a marine base firing my rifle at a target to qualify as a rifleman. I along with others fired at targets three hundred yards distant from where we stood. An officer would walk up and down the firing line and offer suggestions to each of us. He eventually stopped alongside me and offered advise since he felt I might have an opportunity to fire expert. This was a commendation given to a marine who was able to attain a score of 225. I was excited not only by having a chance to fire expert but also that he took an interest in me. As I continued to fire at the target from different positions, he provided suggestions to improve my accuracy. Lo and behold, he informed me that I fired expert...I was thrilled. As I left the firing line, he asked me what I was interested in studying at college. I told him I hadn't decided yet. I then asked about his profession and he told me he was a geologist. Hearing that, I felt this was a special moment. Since I recalled finding a footprint of a dinosaur preserved in shale bed near Holyoke, along with my growing interest in geology, I couldn't let this moment pass. With some excitement, I asked him questions about his work as a geologist, and he responded with similar enthusiasm. As we talked, I began to realize that my interest in geology was quickly growing and I felt this might be my choice for a major. I felt it would work out since I had passed advanced courses in chemistry and math and enjoyed them both. Applying this knowledge to help understand geology was likely to be my next adventure. This person along with others helped put my life on this track and I am forever grateful. Shortly thereafter, I decided to apply for admission to the George Washington University and pursue a degree in geology. The way events happen in people lives that help shape their future can be mysterious.

4

$\mathcal{F}$ollowing My Instincts

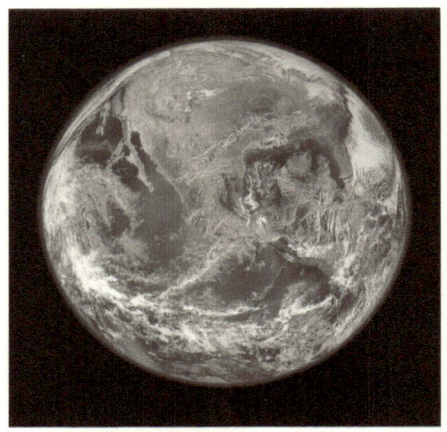

Earth

In the fall of 1964 and while still in the Marine Corps Reserves, I was accepted as an undergraduate at the George Washington University which was located close to where I was living. I was impressed by the name of the university since my birthday, February 22, came on the same day as George Washington's. At the time, it was celebrated as a holiday. It appeared I was destined to attend this university. At this time, I was married and we had two children, a girl and a boy.

The first geology course I registered for was paleontology. The course was to be taught by an instructor who was a paleontologist at the Smithsonian Institution. From the first day of class, I was impressed by his depth of knowledge in the subject as well as other facets of geology. Along with learning much, he also opened my mind to the sciences of biology and geology.

One evening after class, I was asking him a question about his lecture and the subject of fishing was mentioned. As it turned out, we both enjoy fishing, including describing our techniques. He asked me if I would like to go fishing with him sometime. I responded with an enthusiastic yes! We set a date and met at the upper Potomac River.

As we fished, we talked a great deal about geology. I mentioned that I desired a job doing something geological in nature. It was just a few minutes later when he suggested I work for him at the Museum of Natural History. I was excited when I heard his offer, and it only took a moment before I accepted, even before inquiring about the salary. He continued to describe the position and felt the salary would be the same as I received in my current job. This was an opportunity beyond my dreams. I had heard of people getting job offers that closely matched their desires but never felt it would happen to me.

Working at the Smithsonian Institution was an extraordinary experience. I was able to interact with well-educated geologists and listen to their conversations. I could chime in and ask questions, which they gladly responded. While working there, I learned a great deal about what goes into creating the exhibitions for the public to view. I took the time to meet those who did that work and discovered they are a dedicated group who work hard at making exhibits as lifelike as possible. I also met other students like myself, working under the direction of curators, and several were also attending the George Washington University. Since the building I worked in was situated on the Washington Mall, it was convenient to walk to other museum buildings to view exhibits.

The curator was an exceptional geologist and paleontologist. He was my supervisor, instructor, and friend all rolled into one. For me, this was the perfect person to have as a boss. I accompanied him on many fossil-collecting trips within the United States, especially out west in Colorado and Wyoming. This was a great way to learn about geology. We walked and hiked to many locations, even in rainstorms, to collect fossils to be examined after returning to the museum.

After finishing a trip, he gave me the responsibility of cataloging the fossils we collected. While doing this, I observed several similar-looking fossil clams that had been lumped together under one species name, even though they appeared different. When I pointed this out to the curator, he agreed, and we began an exhaustive study of these differences. He finally concluded that these fossils represented three separate species. He eventually published a paper of this study and subsequently gave me credit for recognizing the anatomical differences between these fossil clams. The fossil names as they appeared in the paper were *Thyrasira beauchampi*, *Thyrasira beauchampi beauchampi*, and *Thyrasira beauchampi rex*. I was thrilled that he used my name and considered it an honor. In this field of study, it's very special to have an organism named after an individual.

I continued to work at the Smithsonian Institution until I graduated with a bachelor's degree and began my studies for a master's degree in geology. I soon was offered a position as an oceanographer/geologist at the US Naval Oceanographic Office by a manager who was a part-time instructor at the university. I was being offered a position by someone who knew about me and felt I was qualified. Since this was a permanent position with the U.S. government, I was pleased to accept the offer. It was difficult for me to leave the Smithsonian since I wouldn't be working for my mentor any longer. However, he was my principal adviser for my master's research, and with his guidance, I completed the requirements for the degree. I felt honored when another research geologist read my thesis and informed me the research was superb. A few years later, I became aware that my thesis was used as a reference for students who were taking geology courses at the university. Again, I felt honored.

I made many friends while working for the U.S Navy. Many were experts in various oceanographic disciplines, such as marine biology, atmospheric science, physical oceanography, as well as geology. This combination of various scientific disciplines was the beginning of how scientists began investigating the oceans in earnest. Subjects dealing with the oceans are being integrated with geology and can be taught in one or several courses. I felt privileged to be a part of this coming together of programs to learn more about the oceans of our planet.

When at sea on an oceanographic ship, my daily life was both different and exciting. I performed various investigations, including collecting water samples twenty-four hours a day, along with examining the ocean floor with specialized cameras and seismic equipment. I enjoyed doing my shift very early in the morning while it was still dark, especially when the moon was visible. Its luminescence would be reflected off the tops of waves and partially light up the ship. Since the fantail is near the water surface and where much of the science-related work takes place, I would feel a part of the sea. This might not be too surprising since our entire makeup is largely water, approximating nearly 70 percent.

As an oceanographer, I learned much about the world's oceans and its inhabitants. I was becoming a multi-disciplinary scientist and thoroughly enjoyed it.

5

Terrible News

It was the spring of 1980 and I was living and working in Washington, DC. The last several years had passed quickly and my life had become stale and dismal. The residents were beginning to emerge from their winter shelters and venture outside into the sunlit, warm days. I didn't appreciate this awakening of the spirit in others, especially in me. Changes in the seasons did nothing for my mood. Much of the time I spent recuperating from a hangover and had no desire to be part of an awakening of my spirit. The use of alcohol and cigarettes was beginning to occupy much of my free time, and any desire to maintain a healthy outlook had escaped me a few years earlier. My wife and I had also divorced.

While I still enjoyed my job as an oceanographer/geologist and program manager, I was losing the desire to work diligently. Even though I tended to be creative and strived to develop new approaches to solving problems, I lost much of my self-confidence. At this time, I had been divorced for nearly three years. I had two pre-teenage children, and they were the light of my life. However, I was not doing a good enough job of showing how important they were to me. Deep inside I longed for a sense of fulfillment. Since I had no idea of how to achieve it, I attempted to suppress the yearning.

Along with addictions, I was having relationships with women. Although, I was unaware about what a rewarding and successful relationship should look like. I was not willing to spend the time to discover ways to promote and keep a relationship vibrant. Since

I had very little self-confidence, I couldn't offer qualities that were meaningful. Even though my relationships were transient, they did provide some semblance of a normal life. I became aware that I was running away from myself as well as others. Periodically I would visit my mother in New Jersey. I inherently knew she was my best friend and I could talk to her more frankly than with others. Even so, I felt very much alone and without purpose or direction in my life. Most of the time, I paid very attention to my well- being, however, I did enjoy jogging. I discovered that this relieved me of stress and feelings of tension. When I was in graduate school, I would occasionally jog to reduce anxiety prior to exams.

It was a day like any other when my stepfather called to inform me that my mother had been diagnosed with lung cancer and had become a recluse. He continued to inform me that the cancer was diagnosed as being terminal—at least that's what the doctor told him. He also told me that she wouldn't respond to this news. She had withdrawn from the world and wouldn't communicate with anyone. When I heard this, I felt as though I been struck down. I was confused and would not accept this as absolute fact. I felt I needed to be with her and try to rescue her from this disease. My inner sense told me it was treatable and not necessarily a death knell. Years ago, I tried to save her from an illness by bringing her to a hospital in DC, where she was successfully treated for a much less life-threatening cancer.

After arriving at the hospital where she was admitted, I came to understand the practitioners were intending to allow her to pass away peacefully without doing much to save her. I decided it was up to me to convince her to return with me to Washington, DC, and be admitted to a hospital for treatment. She did communicate with me and after much persuasion agreed to travel and be admitted. She seemed to look forward to coming to D.C. since in the past she would visit me along with my family and care for her grandchildren while I worked. They loved her and always looked forward to her visiting.

As we were leaving to go to Washington, I was warned by the attending nurse to not subject her to heroic attempts to save her life, since there was no hope for survival and it might prolong her suffering. I dismissed the nurse's advice and proceeded to drive there feeling convinced she could be treated. About four hours later, we reached our destination, and I checked her into the hospital and began hoping for the best. A glimmer of hope arose when, following viewing x-ray pictures of her chest, one doctor thought tuberculosis might be the cause of her illness and rapid decline. However, this turned out to be a false hope. The final diagnosis concluded she had terminal lung cancer.

After the first night and following the collapse of one lung she was placed in intensive care. A tube was inserted into her mouth to provide oxygen directly into the lungs. She therefore couldn't speak - she could only move her eyes and head while squeezing my hand. We communicated by these hand squeezes. I would ask a question, and she would respond by squeezing my hand. We hadn't worked out any specific pattern or number of squeezes for communication, but it was better than nothing at all. I felt powerless to do anything to help her and sensed that a vast dark space had come between us.

She was unrecognizable with the plastic tube and mask over her face that provided life-sustaining oxygen. I brought my children to visit her and even though unable to speak, she hugged them and I wept. I felt she suffered terribly and watching this was more than I could bear. Mindful of my own mortality, I would escape by leaving her side. I would return and then leave again. Back and forth I would go until later in the evening I left to return home, anxious to abandon witnessing her agony. She passed away several days later from the cancer that most likely was brought about by many years of smoking cigarettes.

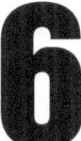

6

$\mathcal{A}$wakening

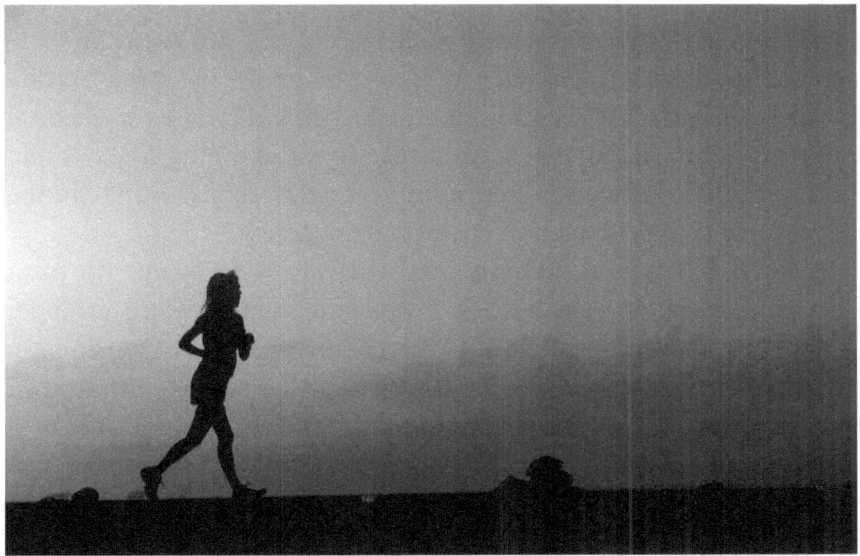

Jogging

Shortly after I learned she had lung cancer, I threw away my cigarettes. To be exact, I flushed them down the toilet; good riddance! While I had tried to stop smoking many times and failed; this time I was determined to quit. I was fearful of getting lung cancer and dying in the same manner. This was a major turning point in my life. To witness her pain, suffering, and eventual death from a disease that is preventable was enough for me to quit smoking.

At first, I found it difficult to stop smoking. I finally managed to quit cold turkey. I was also able to cut back on drinking. When I did drink, I yearned for a cigarette, especially after eating a meal. To relieve this desire, I began chewing straws—small ones, the kind one receives in a mixed drink. Chewing straws was a surrogate for putting a cigarette in my mouth, and it worked.

Along with cutting back on drinking liquor, I was able to avoid smoking altogether. A close friend of mine who was an avid smoker for many years decided to quit with me. His quitting was in deference to my contempt for cigarettes and not wanting to be around smokers while trying to break the habit. He hung in there for about a month. His addiction to nicotine finally overwhelmed his consideration for me, and he began smoking again. I wasn't totally out of the woods, but with every day that I didn't smoke, my resolve to be tobacco free grew stronger.

When I began searching for other ways to keep my mind occupied, I remembered when I was first married and attended college in the evenings, I would jog to relieve feelings of tension and anxiety. Therefore, I began to jog again and discovered that it did help to reduce my anxiety. I also found that it helped me deal with my fears and feelings of guilt. Jogging gave me something positive to think about. I told myself that if I ran, I would not fall victim to the dreaded cancer that infected my mother and brought about her death. That experience made it impossible for me to continue to smoke. The point was to improve my breathing, and I soon realized that smoking was making me short-winded and impaired my ability to sustain jogging for an extended period of time.

Jogging was difficult at first, but in a fairly short time, I began to feel I was getting in shape, and the more I jogged, the better I felt. I continued to jog to keep cigarettes at bay and suppress my feelings of guilt for abandoning my mother. Jogging brought a feeling of freedom and release from my seemingly important and unsurmountable problems. At first, I began with short distances—several times around the park near my apartment. I performed this exercise for specific periods of time; first fifteen minutes, then working up to thirty minutes. I made it a point to jog past my favorite fountain on the senate side of the Capitol Building. At night, this fountain offered a dramatic display of colored lights on cascading streams of water.

Eventually, I began jogging a round trip from Capitol Hill to the Washington Monument. Depending on traffic, this trip would take at least an hour to complete. The route I chose brought me past the U.S. Capitol, down to the Washington Mall, past the buildings that of the Smithsonian Institution, including the Air and Space Museum, the Museum of Natural History, the National Art Gallery, and the History and Technology Building. No longer important was the amount of time I spent jogging. My route had become a tour of the most popular museums in the U.S. Increasing the distance was my goal and soon I was able to extend it beyond the Washington Monument to the Lincoln Memorial. I enjoyed watching tourists marvel at the beauty of the mall. Occasionally I had to avoid running into those who were distracted by all they saw and not paying attention to where they were strolling. Sometimes even I would become distracted to the point of nearly running into a lamppost or a tourist.

If you enjoy watching people, the mall is the place to visit. I would jog past the Vietnam Memorial on my way to the Lincoln Memorial. As I passed that memorial, I felt fortunate to be alive and able to enjoy the pleasure of being outside and exercising. I felt a great sadness for all those who lost their lives in that conflict. I possibly served with some in my earlier life as a marine reservist. Soon after I heard reports about marines killed in a terrorist bombing of their barracks in Beirut, I jogged to the Washington Monument. I stared at the circle of American flags surrounding it and wished those marines could have been with me to feel the fresh and free air that surrounded me—the same air they were dedicated to protect. I became overcome with sadness and wept. I continue to experience the same emotion when I think about their dedication to our country and to all of us.

I wasn't the only person running on the mall. This is a favorite route for fitness addicts in Washington. The mall is an all-season route for joggers, bikers, and also strollers. The fall and summer months are the best times for outdoor enjoyment. Winters are not all bad except for occasional storms or blizzards, which can hinder the most dedicated joggers. However, there are those who will still venture out to jog in any kind of weather. I have jogged both in the rain and following a snowstorm when the paths and sidewalks were cleared; but I didn't make it a standard practice. In fact, I would advise against it. Taking several days off until storms cease and the roads and sidewalks are totally clear will not, in my opinion, result in one losing any amount of fitness. We all need to be careful about being too compulsive.

When I began running, I found evenings to be the best time, particularly in the summer when it's the coolest part of the day. I enjoyed seeing how the shadows from buildings and lampposts fell across the mall. When it rains, the light from street lights highlight the raindrops and give a surreal appearance. When on the return trip from the Washington Monument to Capitol Hill, I was able take in the splendor of the Capitol building at the west side of the mall. In the evenings, the Capitol would be ablaze with light from floodlights. At this writing, floodlights are no longer used on the mall since they can be a distraction to planes landing at the nearby Ronald Reagan Airport in Virginia.

My body was beginning to respond positively to the rigor I was putting it through. In those times, I ran nearly every night. The night air felt good against my face. Occasionally, when it was misty or even raining, the moisture that fell on me was refreshing and made me feel acutely aware that I was alive. I would concentrate on listening to my breathing. It might be forced at first, then would become more relaxed, uniform, and less strained. When I jogged during the day, the sunlight warmed me on cool days, and on warm or hot days perspiration would cause my clothes to stick to my skin. This perspiration was a reminder of having a good workout. Running gave me that high many people have felt and talked about. It's a feeling of lightness and alertness I had not often experienced. At times I ran with abandonment, eager to feel my prowess and discover my full potential. Other times I concentrated more on the surrounding environment, i.e., the trees along the mall, water in the reflecting pool, birds and squirrels as they scampered along the ground and in the trees. Many of the birds were seagulls seemingly seeking a new home away from water. I often wondered if any were aware of their ocean heritage. Maybe they completely acclimated to an existence near the mall and the reflecting pool waiting for scraps of food from passing tourists. I rather hoped they were just passing by and paying a visit.

Running is an excellent way to increase the ability of our respiratory system to function well and increase our stamina. However, it's not always practical or possible. As much as I may enjoy jogging in a warm rain, I certainly don't enjoy being caught in a torrential downpour; and it has happened. It may also be too warm or the local air conditions may be such that just breathing may be injurious to one's health. A good example is emissions from cars and trucks, especially in areas of heavy traffic. Some runners place bandanas on their faces to trap emission particles before being taken into their lungs. I have seen photos of people in China wearing bandanas on their faces to prevent them from breathing polluted air. Whether this can help prevent lung disease is up for debate and beyond the scope of this book.

Recently on a trip with my wife to Cairo, Egypt to visit her bother, I decided to jog on streets near to where he lived. I was quite excited about this venture since I wanted to see a bit of Cairo from a jogger's viewpoint. The streets were congested with traffic and I would jog across them quickly when it stopped for some reason. As I continued to run, I saw people sitting most anywhere eating food since Ramadan had recently ended. I continued to run to and around a rundown-looking racetrack. I later discovered it was used for horse racing at an earlier time. Many who saw me didn't seem to pay much attention. I assumed they had witnessed others doing the same along the streets or were just too involved with celebrating the end of Ramadan. Apart from dealing with the heavy traffic, jogging can be a reasonable way to tour Cairo provided you're familiar with the area and don't lose your way.

7

$\mathcal{F}$itness While Vacationing

In 1981 my father passed away after a long illness—one year following the death of my mother. I felt depressed and hoping to change my mood, I decided to go abroad and tour Europe. As I packed my bag, I decided to jog in those countries I visited. I packed running shorts, T-shirts, and sneakers while being excited about jogging in foreign countries. This seemed a novel way to go on tour and I'm not aware of a description of this manner in any travel literature.

After arriving in London and recovering from jet lag, I put on my jogging clothes and set out on the street. As I ran, many people turned to gaze at me with some wonderment. I didn't feel they had experienced many people jogging along their thoroughfares. I continued through several beautiful parks and squares. When I passed through Trafalgar Square the residing pigeons took flight, much to the dismay of tourists feeding them. As I continued, I could cover a significant amount of territory. While I may have been viewed as an oddity, many would offer friendly waves or pleasant nods. It was a wonderful experience as I jogged by well-known places in London, such as Buckingham Palace.

I decided to take the train to visit Westminster Abbey. When I arrived, it was windy and sunny and the residents were wearing dark robes while having trouble keeping them on. It was quite amusing to watch both students and faculty struggling to prevent their robes from blowing away. They looked like huge blackbirds flapping in the wind as they hurried along. I strolled around the grounds of the abbey and viewed ancient-looking memorials at various locations. Jogging didn't appear appropriate, so instead I walked around the outside of the church several times to view its entirety.

When I arrived in Paris by train the next evening, I proceeded to check into my hotel near the Eiffel Tower. I decided that when I woke the next morning, I would jog over to view it. I felt excited since I had seen many pictures of the tower and now I was going to finally view it.

The October morning was bright, sunny, and cool and I hurried to put on my jogging clothes. I didn't stop for breakfast and in my exuberance, bolted out of the hotel onto the street almost knocking over two people. I could only imagine what they hollered at me in French as I ran down the street. After an early morning rain shower, the sidewalks leading to the Eiffel Tower were slick. I could feel my heart beating fast with excitement. As I glanced upward, I could see the top of the tower.

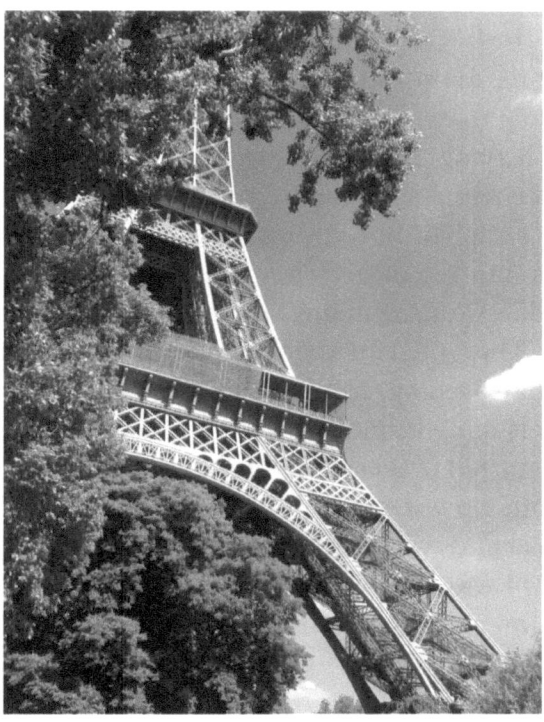

I decided I would proceed down the long axis of the mall toward government buildings without viewing the entire structure until I would turn and run toward the tower. As I ran past government buildings, I was filled with anticipation in seeing this edifice that so epitomized Paris. I also noticed how similar the Paris mall is to the Smithsonian Mall in Washington, DC.

When I finally reached the end of the mall and turned to run back, the entire Eiffel Tower came into full view. I was ecstatic! It appeared majestic, rising upward into the clear blue morning sky. I saw people at different levels enjoying the view. I jogged up to and under the tower, waving as I passed. Many waved back and shouted acknowledgments—mostly in French but some in languages I couldn't identify, much less understand. They all seemed to be smiling and some cheering….I assumed they were supportive. I suddenly realized I was the only jogger in sight.

While in Paris, I also ran along the River Seine and past the Arc de Triumph and down the Champs Elysees. It was a marvelous visual experience…, again I didn't see others exercising along the route I chose. In 1981, jogging didn't appear to be popular in Paris. When seeing me many onlookers appeared a bit puzzled, however, all were willing to extend a wave or a smile as I passed.

Prior to leaving Paris, I visited Notre Dame church in the evening. As I entered the church, there were several visitors sitting or kneeling. I slipped into a pew and kneeled to pray. It wasn't long before a number of people arrived and began gathering near a piano. I realized that it might be the choir coming in to rehearse their music. They filed in together like my choir in D.C. does every Thursday evening. It wasn't long before they began to sing. The music was quite beautiful, and as I knelt, I thought about my parents and started to weep. I'm not sure how long I wept. A man sitting in front slowly stood up, turned, and put a hand on my shoulder. His hand was reassuring and caring, and I was grateful for his touch. I was happy to be in another country listening to a choir with similar musical abilities as other choirs in the world coming together to rehearse their music. I was both at awe and saddened.

When I finally arrived in Switzerland by train, my plan was to visit Zermatt. I soon discovered that jogging wasn't practical or advantageous in this area since getting around requires walking mostly uphill or downhill. I decided to concentrate my energies on walking and hiking. Admittedly this was a bit slower, although it was very rewarding especially in a setting like Zermatt. The Swiss Alps rise majestically around Zermatt with the Matterhorn standing in bold relief. Fortunately, I had increased my ability to hike by exercising and could walk for long distances and at high altitudes without tiring out. This was a benefit I hadn't anticipated. There was much to see on the trails and footpaths and I could get close to nature and view wildlife.

Much later, I vacationed at Mt. Rainier in the state of Washington to view and hike on mountain trails. After a day of getting used to the altitude and time change, I found myself able to hike many of the trails with quite a bit of exuberance. Fortunately, I had enough energy left over to sit before a fireplace in the hotel and share with others the high points of my day's adventure. I recall thinking that years earlier I wouldn't have been able to engage in this venture and likely would have quit early on and head for the so-called barn to recuperate. There was so much to see and I discovered other trails to different parts of the mountain. If I wanted to enjoy the wide and beautiful vistas of the Cascade Range I would have to hike up to the high trails. When I took on this challenge, I was surprised to see people who were older than me. One senior-looking person informed me that every year he looked forward to coming here. His plan was to keep fit so he could continue to hike into this high country and enjoy the spectacular views and wildlife. I hadn't realized it at first, but exercising had prepared me to hike for fairly long periods of time and at high altitudes.

There is a lake in Pennsylvania, where in the past several years, I feel fortunate to visit in the summer with my wife. The days are mostly cool and bright, and when sunlight is reflected off the water, it sparkles. With a dog occasionally beside me, I would jog or walk around the lake, taking in the splendor of the hemlock and pine trees that proliferate the area. As usual, I would feel in touch with the surroundings. Being able to easily hike into areas like this to enjoy the beauty and swim in cool turbulent streams are rewards for being fit.

Once on a trip to Aiken, South Carolina, I stayed overnight in nearby Augusta, Georgia, and took advantage of jogging along a path adjacent to the Savannah River. This river marks the border between South Carolina and Georgia. It was in the early evening, and the scenery was spectacular. The river sparkled as the sun's rays reflected off the water. The air felt fresh and cool as the wind blew across the river toward me. As often happens when jogging or walking quickly, my senses of sight and smell are sharp and I'm able to appreciate the environment.

Another time in the distant past, when I traveled to San Francisco on a business trip, I took the opportunity to jog in the city. I left my hotel in early morning with a plan to go to Seal Rock. This is a location in the bay where a large number of seals congregate on large near-shore rocks and their barking can be heard from quite a distance. Jogging there is a terrific scenic experience since it took me through well-known parts of the city as well as areas that were at the time depressed. After arriving, I marveled at the sights and sounds of seals swimming, barking, and reclining on rocks close to shore. After returning to the hotel, I felt my round-trip jog was worthwhile since I toured a good part of the city, viewed a large number of seals, and had a great exercise. Again, it appeared I was the only person jogging and was occasionally viewed with astonishment.

8

The Atlanta 10K

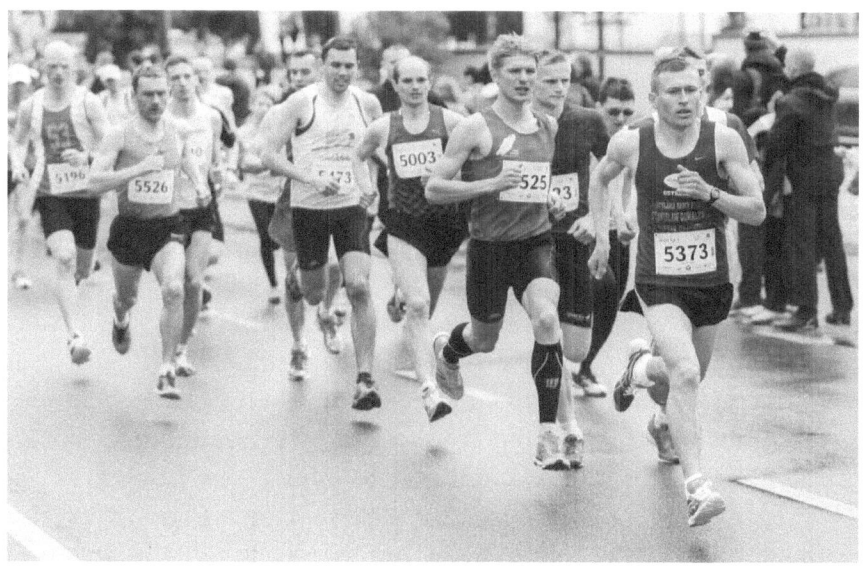

When I lived and worked in Atlanta in 1992-1995, jogging continued to be an important part of my routine. I found that jogging through upscale neighborhoods was quite scenic. Since some residents had dogs, it was best to hurry through those areas and not attract their attention. While living there, I decided to participate in the Atlanta 10K race. This is a celebrated event in Atlanta. The race takes place on July 4th when the temperature can be close to one hundred degrees; a little cooler if fortune smiles upon you. It begins in the northern part of the city called Buckhead and continues down Peachtree Street and ends at Piedmont Park in midtown Atlanta.

After hearing about this event, I decided to participate. It turned out the experience was one I will never forget. Along with others, I made my way to the starting line by subway. Many were dressed in the most colorful running outfits I had ever seen. To stand out in the crowd seemed to be the objective.

The subway was filled to overflowing and the excitement was contagious; almost overwhelming. I never had a more fun-filled ride on a subway. When we arrived, I was surprised to see mobs of people mingling around the starting line. Large groups were being formed and I was told by a female runner, who was more knowledgeable about this race than I was, that the race begins by allowing one group to proceed, followed by another group a few minutes later. In that way, we don't get bunched up into an incredible knot of humanity somewhere along the route. I discovered later that nearly fifty thousand runners participated in this 10K. The object of the race is not necessarily to win but to finish while having the time of your life along the way. There were professional runners who would start early and finish before the first group of us were allowed to proceed down Peachtree Street.

All of us who embarked from the subway were herded into a group along with other excited people, soon to be runners of the 1993 race. There were volunteers who had the chore of forming up the groups along with keeping our spirits up by telling us how great an event this is. We didn't need much inspiration since the hype was incredibly high. As I stood in my group waiting for the go-ahead from one of the volunteers, my stomach was experiencing the butterfly syndrome. I tried to keep busy by stretching and talking with other runners. After watching the groups ahead of us get the go ahead, we finally received our wave on, and away we went. We jogged slow at first to get the feel of the road and to relax. The route winds down Peachtree Street, past midtown, and finally into the park.

The excitement was truly contagious. For the first quarter-mile I didn't feel the pavement under my feet and I felt light as a feather.

There were many water stations along the way where one could grab a cup of water, gulp it down or spill it over one's head. As we continued down Peachtree Street, we passed several restaurants and bars where customers had ventured out to see us pass. Some even offered us beer or a mixed drink. Water trucks were outfitted with hoses that provided a water spray, which cascaded down upon us as we passed by. There were moments when I felt I was taking a shower. After about a mile, I began to feel the heat. Luckily, it was a partly cloudy day. Although, when the sun came out, I felt I was being broiled alive. I gulped down water at every station and poured it over my head. At one point, behind me I heard a cadence being called in a group of about twelve men from a military academy. In only a few moments they caught up to me. They were being led by a person carrying a brightly colored banner. I felt rejuvenated by their cadence and was able to keep up with them for a short while. They soon outpaced me and I enviously watched them pass out of sight as I listened to their cadence for as long as possible.

Another time when I needed to be revitalized occurred when I was running down one of the many hills in Atlanta and saw ahead of me, high above the street, a man on a latter holding a camera. He was waving at me to look up so he could take a picture. My ego prompted me to straighten up and look determined to finish the race. After all, since I was on camera, I needed to look good! Shortly after the race, I received the photo in my mail and it remains one of my prized possessions.

As we began to near Piedmont Park, onlookers shouted encouragement as we passed. I felt buoyed by their shouting and I knew I would finish. We finally turned off Peachtree Street and headed down a side street toward the park. Ahead I could see the finish line and runners walking off into the park. Before long a person told me that I completed the race and could go and pick up my T-shirt. I had forgotten that my badge of courage for finishing the 10K was the shirt. Once I saw others wearing theirs, it took me no time in getting to the tables where they were available and claim my own. That shirt is still part of my wardrobe and I proudly wear it on July 4, when I can find it in my chest of drawers.

Successfully finishing the race gave me the incentive to keep up with jogging. It was a great way to keep my weight under control. Since I also discovered that my appetite had increased, I needed to be certain I didn't gain too much weight. I frequently jogged in midtown Atlanta past many beautiful homes. Many streets were laced with tall trees and flourishing shrubs. In the spring, it was difficult to be attentive to where I was heading since the flowers were abundant, colorful, and their diversity was magnificent. One street was especially enjoyable since many of the houses were mansions and were well kept. Atlanta tends to be hilly, so I was continually tested to jog up and down without slowing down too much.

I will elaborate more later on about my experiences while living and working in Atlanta.

9

Working Out

Running or jogging can be more than just exercise. For some, it can be as important as water, food, and sleep. Although for me, it had not reached that level of importance. I looked forward to being outside and allow my spirit to take control and guide my legs over the ground. I also added exercising on machines in fitness centers and reduced the number of days I jogged.

At the recreation center in the Department of the Interior in D.C. where I was once employed in the 1980's, I had joined the recreation center and was among the first to sign up. I spent a lot of my time playing racquetball and basketball with friends and we all became quite skilled. Since I didn't find this fulfilling, I decided to try working out on the exercise machines. At first, the machines were intimidating and I didn't wish to look foolish using them. I also had doubts they would help increase my strength and fitness. These were not the more popular ones that were advertised, but as I started using them, they were challenging and provided a good workout.

The workout room was small but adequate. My living and dining area's combined were about the same size. The room reminded me of the inside of a railroad car, long and narrow, with exercise machines lined up along both sides of the room facing each other. Even though no mirrors were available where one could inspect their technique, I could observe someone on the other side of the room as I was on a machine. This might have been embarrassing, so I tried to keep my eyes trained straight ahead.

After receiving instructions and an exercise program from the fitness instructor, I went at it full tilt. This was different from the type of exercising I was familiar with since it stressed exercising different body parts (i.e., legs, arms, and back). Over time, I began to feel the impact on my musculature from this more focused method. When I finished working out my body seemed to tingle and I felt aglow with energy. However, when I woke the following morning, I felt the pain associated with exercising muscles that had not been fully stressed before. This can be a crucial time for anyone who wishes to become fit; to either keep at it or quit.

For some, the experience of feeling pain can result in not wanting to continue and one may drop out of a fitness program. For example, the following arguments might be used to refrain from exercising: One might complain, "This is too painful" or "I can hardly move the next day" or "I'm probably too old to do this sort of thing anyway." Many older people and even seniors seem to agree that advanced age can prevent them from participating in strenuous activities. This is especially true if we've been told that as you grow older you should do less, relax more and not stress yourself. This focus on age is likely to prevent many from exercising. I am not aware of anyone who has demonstrated that advanced age is a major deterrent to exercising. Illness yes, but not necessarily age. The two are not necessarily synonymous. Medical evidence is beginning to suggest many benefits can result from exercising and becoming fit. It is commonly understood that it can add muscle and help strengthen our bodies, including heart, arms, back, stomach, and legs. Additionally, bone strengthening may be a benefit and help prevent osteoporosis. Doctors may inform you that if you're healthy enough to exercise, by all means do it, but be sure to follow instructions from a professional trainer. Early on I had a physical exam, and after receiving an electrocardiogram, my doctor informed me that my heart action was similar to that of a long-distance runner. That was very satisfying to hear and made me feel I had accomplished something significant for myself.

About six months after I began exercising, I became aware of changes in my body. My biceps, chest and even my legs muscles become large. I felt stronger and I also kept up with jogging. I would jog at least twice during the week and once on the weekend; preferably Sunday morning. It's my opinion that just getting out there and exercising, we all stand a better chance of being around for a much longer time. This is the time to enjoy our lives and our children, grandchildren, and friends. We all have so much to offer the world, so why should we deprive it and ourselves?

Nowadays there are very good fitness centers or gyms to choose from. Some are well organized and offer many options, including aerobic classes, exercise machines, free weights, tennis, swimming, racquetball; the list goes on and on. A fitness center that offers several options to exercising is my preference. At the very least, attending aerobic classes, walking quickly, using exercise machines, and exercising limbs with weights are generally required. It is important to feel comfortable with the physical setting of the fitness center and the kind of clientele that attend. The attitude of trainers is also important. They need to be courteous, helpful, mindful of our physical limitations, and trained in administering assistance. The success of each workout can largely depend on the guidance received from the trainers.

10

$\mathcal{B}$onding and Support

Ideveloped close friendships at fitness centers when living in Atlanta and elsewhere. These friendships were important as sources of encouragement. Today, they have the same importance and even more so as I continue to exercise. I discovered that those who exercise together and assist each other develop a nurturing relationship. A strong bond can be formed at a level not likely experienced in casual meetings with others. This may be similar to the way athletes on the same team bond with each other.

In my forties and nearly the same today, my routine at the gym consisted of exercising my upper body two days a week and lower body two days a week. I also jogged or did other aerobic exercise as well. I would rest on Saturday and Sunday. If the weather cooperated, I might jog on Sundays. I was forty-six years old at the time, and feeling great.

At that time, my office in the Department of the Interior was being transferred to California and I was offered the opportunity to relocate and assist in managing a technical program. Since I had little desire to move away from my children, I decided to resign and apply to graduate school to earn a PhD in geology.

During this time, exercising became even more important. This physical activity helped me from losing confidence and zeal to earn a PhD degree. The loss of job and returning to school both took a toll on my psyche. My anxiety level shot up about 1,000 percent and I felt I lost part of my identity and was mentally floundering. Exercise did offer me relief from a good deal of frustration and anxiety, although not all. To find relief, I would often go to the gym and exercise. This is when free weights became part of my workout routine. In the past, I would primarily use barbells for working out my biceps. However, I had not attempted bench-pressing or other kinds of exercises with free weights. Those weights were just not available in the other places where I exercised.

The PhD program in geology turned out to be a fulfilling experience as I learned more about both geology and oceanography, along with interacting with professors and other graduate students. To become aware about advances in the geosciences was both stimulating and rewarding along with making new friends among my peers and also participating in departmental functions. I began to realized I was attracted to the idea of working in academia as a professor and felt it might be the best role for me in future years.

My relationship with my children took a significant turn for the better. I had more time for them, and I wasn't feeling sorry for myself. I felt better and had more energy. I began taking my son for long bike rides that became a great way to tour Washington. Then, at a much later time, he along with his wife and their three-year-old daughter began biking in a serious way. I also started taking my son skiing. A sport I felt I would never take up in my fifties. He appeared to get the hang of it quickly. My ability to communicate with both my son and daughter improved to the point where they could tell me how they felt when their mother and I were divorced. It was difficult for me to hear, but healing for them to tell me. I feel exercising relieved me of those inhibitions that prevented me from being there for them. Guilt no longer motivated me to stay away. I could tell them how much I loved them and that I was always available. I feel that when you feel good about yourself, this attitude comes naturally. When I didn't feel that way, I hid and didn't want them to see how unsure I was of myself.

Upon completing the PhD and celebrating this accomplishment, I took a management position offered to me in 1992 that was located in Atlanta, Georgia. I was hired to manage the cleaning up of waste landfill sites that were closed due to hazardous materials being buried there. This was a challenge since even though I had earned a doctorate degree, I had a lot to learn about waste landfill sites and the kinds of contamination that can be released and impact surrounding environments.

One of the first things I did after arriving in Atlanta was to locate a fitness center. I found one almost immediately. The center had every exercise machine known to the modern world and included weights for lifting exercises, racquetball, swimming, and even included mirrors on the walls. At first, I felt conspicuous and a bit hesitant to use these mirrors. Once I overcame my shyness, I was able to benefit from using various exercise machines. With mirrors, I could critique my technique and adjust my positions to prevent possible injury. Mirrors provided opportunities to watch myself and others to learn proper techniques. There was the advantage of ignoring pain or discomfort by admiring the opposite sex engaged in doing their routines.

After joining the center, I immediately began working out even before I found a permanent place to live. In time and with encouragement from the resident staff, I began bench-pressing with free weights. I was very cautious at first. I watched others as they lifted weights and the various exercises they used. When I finally began lifting weights, it hurt at first; in fact, it hurt quite a bit. I began following the advice from trainers to go slow. It took several months before my body became accustomed with this method of exercising and in fact I began to feel stronger.

I became friendly with a man who I later discovered was sixty-three years old and an avid athlete. He consistently exercised and most every time I was there, he was present. He provided me advice and I listened closely to what he had to recommend. I attempted to incorporate some of his suggestions into my workout. For a period of time, he became my mentor. While I received good instructions from trainers at the facility, I relied on his coaching and suggestions since he was older and closer to my age and life experiences. I wanted to be very cautious about whose advice I followed. I didn't want to do anything harmful and therefore desired suggestions from someone with experience. Later I was informed he was an active participator in the Senior Olympics. This type of Olympics is for seniors over fifty years old. People must qualify for the event they wish to compete in by presenting a document of qualification for the same competitive event they accomplished during the past year.

Sharing and mutual understanding often occur in the gym. When you ask a trainer or someone else to spot you in a lift, that person generally understands what you're requesting. He or she is aware of your need and will normally respond to assist you. They may or may not voice their support, but a nod of the head is generally enough of a response. A bond between the lifter and spotter may often be formed. The lifter trusts that the spotter will assist if their strength fails in the middle of a lift. Except for the military, enforcement, and safety occupations, this kind of trust is rarely experienced in other kinds of situations. Responding to the needs of another person without knowing them is a benefit. This response to such a need seems a part of being human. I frequently placed my safety in the hands of others in the fitness room, and never was I disappointed. The exercise room is a place where people generally won't walk away from your need. My friend frequently encouraged me to do a little more. He was also there to rescue me from being overly optimistic. In my opinion, this kind of encouragement and assistance is critical in completing a successful workout.

My relationship with my children took a turn for the better. I had more time for them, and I wasn't feeling sorry for myself. I felt better and had more energy. I began taking my son for long bike rides that became a great way to tour Washington. I also started taking my son skiing. A sport I felt I would never take up in my fifties. He appeared to get the hang of it quickly. My ability to communicate with both my son and daughter improved to the point where they could tell me how they felt when their mother and I were divorced. It was difficult for me to hear, but healing for them to tell me. I feel exercising relieved me of those inhibitions that prevented me from being there for them. Guilt no longer motivated me to stay away. I could tell them how much I loved them and that I was always available. I feel that when you feel good about yourself, this attitude comes naturally. When I didn't feel that way, I hid and didn't want them to see how unsure I was of myself.

$\mathcal{V}$arying My Routine

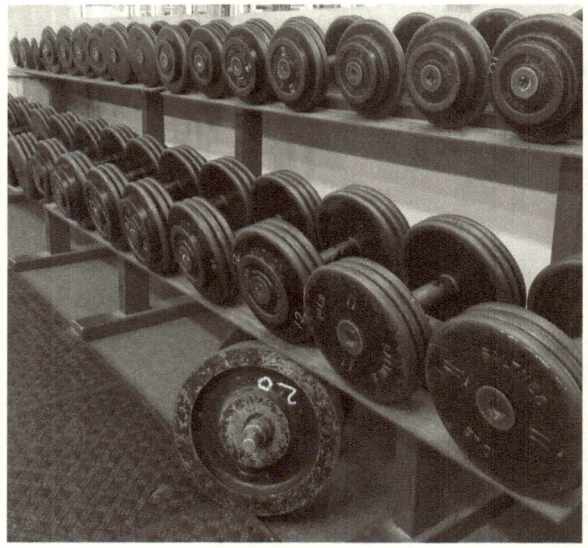

Weight Lifting

While I continued to work out on exercise machines, I added weight lifting to my routine. I focused on using bench-pressing to exercise my chest and arms: five sets with about eight to ten repetitions per set. This consisted of less weight and a higher number of repetitions for the first set; increasing the weight and less repetitions for the second set; and even less weight and increased repetitions toward the end. This is what trainers call pyramiding. I performed this routine when exercising my biceps, triceps, and shoulders. For my lower body, I used the same routine, but I used machines instead of individual weights. Incorporating weights into my routine was beneficial and was difficult to be duplicated with other types of exercises. Exercising with weights added new challenges to my workout.

In deciding on the amount of weight to use during any exercise, I thought about the extent I wished to push myself and how I felt physically. As previously stated, I began with weights I could handle easily. I would continue to add more weight until I pushed myself to lift nearly the maximum amount of weight. When I placed weights on the bar, I would try to visualize the lift and prepare myself for the exertion. Lying on the bench, I would grasp the bar with both hands and position them far enough apart to feel comfortable. I then concentrated on lifting the bar and weights upward. I would feel the heaviness through both my arms and chest. Then I allowed the bar to sink down toward my chest, and just before it touched, I would again lift upward, extending my arms to full extension. At the same time, I inhaled when the bar was descending to my chest and exhaled when I lifted. This procedure would hopefully prevent me from forcing too much blood throughout my body and prevent a possible rupture. I repeated these lifts until my strength was nearly depleted. I would repeat these exercises three to five times (or sets) with about six to eight repetitions in each set.

Occasionally I might make strange-sounding noises while lifting weights and would try to avoid worrying if anyone could hear me. I began to feel good about what I could accomplish and periodically would attempt to add a bit more weight to my routine. I began to fully understand my limits to take on more weight. As time passed, I felt stronger. I didn't mind being alone in the gym, and many times I preferred it. When I went to bed at night, my body occasionally ached from the exercise. Stretching would help lessen the aches. By afternoon, it had mostly disappeared and I felt I was adapting to the exercise.

12

Changes in Me

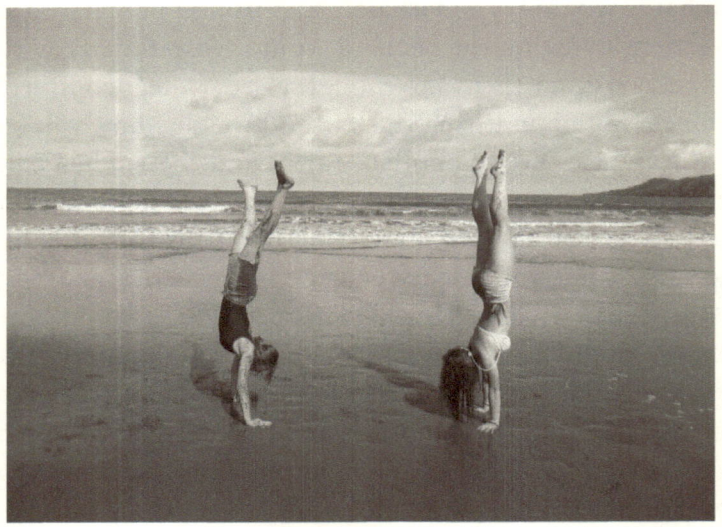

Aerobics

I have frequently asked myself, what is it that begins to change in me when I exercise regularly? This can be difficult to explain. Many people probably exercise to look physically attractive. That doesn't totally explain what is going on with me. The Greeks, especially the Spartans, recognized the importance of a healthy mind in a healthy body. This concept impressed me and has been one of my guiding principles for becoming fit. When exercising

I can concentrate on issues and derive solutions to problems much faster. My mind is clearer, and my perspective about myself improved. After a few years, I discovered more about who I am. This was an important time for me, and I feel it promoted maturity. Understanding the workings of my body, including being in touch with my abilities, was important to me. When I was not in good shape, my senses were somewhat blurred. When I was fit, I was more aware of my existence in the world, at least from a physical perspective. My life began to take on new meanings. The strength and endurance I gained through working out was my reward, albeit fleeting. I breathed easily; food and drink tasted good; I could think clearly; I worked faster; I smiled easier and longer; and I felt better about myself, which was a huge step forward in my life.

We all want to look the best we can, but is that the main force for exercising? Is that what pushed me to exercise four or five days a week, even while on vacation? I feel the principal reason why I continued this schedule then and even now, is to prepare myself to deal with living my life. This often involves dealing with disappointments, failures, loss, depression, and even successes. I am currently able to take disappointments and letdowns easier. Feeling depressed doesn't stay with me as long as it did prior to exercising. Finding solutions to issues tend to be easier.

Unfortunately, while this happens to many of us; my wife and I were not getting along, so we decided to separate. This separation created a great deal of stress and anxiety in my life. There were times when I felt like giving up in attempting to carry on with my career or taking on new challenges. Again, consistently exercising helped me to remain positive about my life. It also provided me with something important to concentrate on while I was going through the grieving process. Additionally, exercising gave me the resolve and spirit to remain fit. This required me to eat and sleep regularly. Since alcohol is a detriment to good physical conditioning, I was not tempted to overindulge. Regular exercise helped to keep me focused on what was important and not give in to destructive behaviors like taking drugs or smoking cigarettes.

As can happen, there were times when I felt too tired to

exercise. If I didn't feel up to it, I might try to convince myself to lay off. However, instead of giving into this temptation, this was an important time to do some sort of exercise. As it turns out, when I do exercise, I feel refreshed. I may have to push myself a bit harder to break through a period of feeling lazy. When I finish a workout, I feel good about myself for not giving into the temptation of avoidance.

To be in the gym provides opportunities to concentrate on what the body is experiencing. It is uplifting to be in touch with one's body, especially when your breathing is deep and regular, your heart is beating strongly, and perspiration is dripping from your pores. This is part of the reward for exercising and may also include feeling strong, alert, confident, yet also meditative. It's an overall experience that can add much pleasure to our lives. It can also be very personal, although there is immense pleasure in sharing the experience with others.

$\mathscr{R}$eturning to the Gym

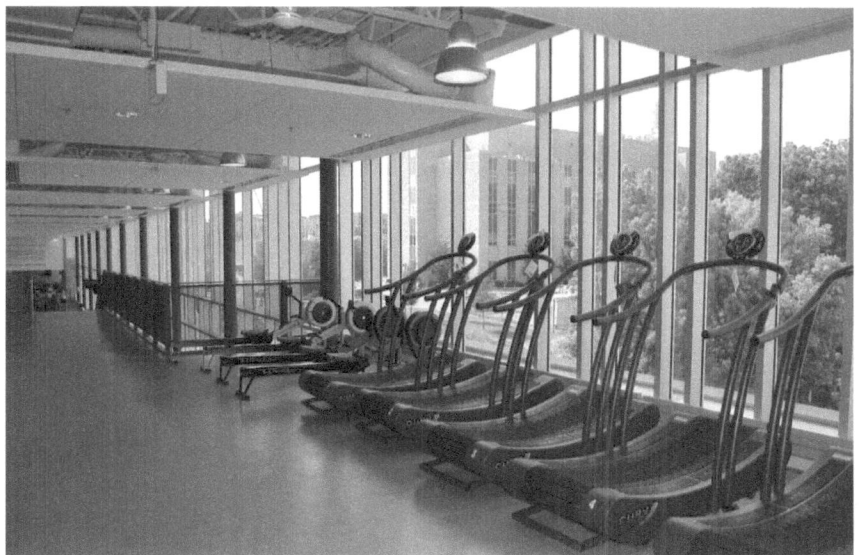

The Gym

In late 1992, I had returned to Washington, DC, to take a position to teach and be the director of a graduate degree program in environmental management at the University of Maryland University College. This was the type of position I had hoped for since receiving my PhD. Since there is no lack of fitness centers and places to jog in the area, I felt in my element. This was one of the selling points of the job, even though I was thrilled to become part of academia. As stated earlier, I had wanted to teach since I first decided to become a geologist along with my experiences working as one.

As I did when arriving in Atlanta, I signed up at the university gym and began to work out at my normal pace of four to five days a week, alternating jogging and upper and lower body exercises. I used two different workout areas in the gym—one area that had exercise machines, including step machines for aerobics and another small area that contained only free weights. This small area had recently been built, and I reverently coined it my sweat room. I enjoyed jogging on the running track around the university football stadium. I was fortunate in making friends, especially where I would frequently exercise and also those who offered assistance or advice.

Early on I learned that injuries may occur if I'm not careful when exercising. When this occurred, I would reduce my workouts by slowing down while jogging, using lighter weights, or just stop working out entirely until I felt better. Occasionally, I would continue with reduced aerobic exercises until I was completely healed. Later-on I elaborate more on this issue.

14

$\mathcal{A}$ Close Call

In the summer of 1995, I went to a beach on the coast of Virginia with my fiancée, to enjoy the sun and surf and see the well-known wild ponies. It was a beautiful Labor Day weekend; the temperature was warm, and the surf was strong. Offshore storms and a distant hurricane resulted in the surf being quite high, and their frequency of occurrence was rapid. Reports of riptides, where water flows back from the beach into the ocean resulting in strong undertows, were numerous and there were several reported in the general area.

Over the entire weekend, we had been swimming outside of the surf zone in deep water. I enjoyed floating on top of the waves and looking up at the sky. On the last day before returning to Washington, we decided to swim again for the last time. Once we were outside of the near-shore breakers, the water was good for swimming, although there were large swells that buoyed us over incoming waves. Without realizing it, we were quickly carried offshore by a riptide. I shouted to my companion that we should swim back to shore. At that moment, a large wave broke over us. I felt myself being spun around and pushed deeply downward into the water, spinning as I descended. My right arm was violently jerked backward by the increased water pressure from the wave. This contorted movement resulted in the separation of my shoulder. I felt pain shoot down my entire arm, but I still retained feeling in it. Realizing I was injured, I kept swimming toward shore. Even though my shoulder felt separated, I could partially use the arm for swimming by holding it on the water surface to balance myself while I stroked feverishly with my left arm. Several times I caught a glimpse of blue sky and scattered white clouds that appeared detached from my situation. This beauty appeared to be discordant with what was going on with me. I felt rushes of fear that caused me to shake as I swam. Smaller waves broke over me, but I was able to keep myself on the surface. The water as it rushed shoreward gently stroked my face as it passed. It felt like a caress reassuring me I would be fine. I felt that if I were to drown, it would be a beautiful day to end my existence on earth. I suppressed these thoughts and focused my attention and strength on swimming to shore while encouraging my companion to keep heading toward shore. I hoped my strength would sustain me until I reached land. I finally found myself unceremoniously washed up onto the beach on the seat of my bathing suit. As I stood up, a couple sitting on the beach gave me a thumbs-up. I felt like Jonah after being vomited by the sea onto the shore.

As I picked myself out of the surf, I could not straighten my right arm. I realized it was separated and I had come close to drowning in that turbulent water. I found our blanket on the beach and along with my companion, I collapsed. I realized that my strength and endurance saved me from losing the struggle. Before this experience, I used to wonder whether I would ever be called upon to use whatever strength I gained through exercise. I don't wonder any longer; it happened and may again sometime. Doctors managed to reset my shoulder, and I could return to work. I had to wear an arm sling until it was healed. The path back to fitness remained in front of me and became another challenge.

15

The Road Back, Again

I did begin working out again, albeit slowly. At first, I attempted to bench-press only the bar with no weights on it. As the days passed, I added a small amount of weight and began lifting with my left arm. It was painful when I put strain or stress on my right arm and shoulder. However, each time I entered the fitness room, I wanted to perform a little better than I had the previous time.

During that period, it didn't seem I was making much progress. About four months later, I was back lifting weights. Difficult as it was, I felt I was making progress. I could bench-press more than half the weight I could before the accident, and my arm strength was improving at about the same rate. I felt I was finally beginning to return to where I was physically prior to the injury. Although I realized I could easily reinjure myself again. Therefore, I maintained a constant slow level of improvement. I found that stretching my arm and shoulder with different exercises prescribed by medical doctors at the university helped me to mend. By slowly adding weight to the barbells and having patience, It took nearly a year to gain back the fitness I had lost. If I hadn't been fit when I received the injury, it probably would have been much longer before I regained my strength. As I progressed, I felt stiffness in my shoulder, although this was reduced when I would first stretch both my arm and shoulder. I realized I would likely feel some stiffness there for the rest of my life. It's not an obstacle, only a reminder that I'm human and thus vulnerable.

My efforts to regain fitness helped me in other aspects of my life, including work as a college professor and administrator. I was able to focus on important issues about teaching and develop strategies to deal with them. The road back while difficult, I did receive much encouragement from relatives, friends and co-workers. I didn't realize it then, but years later I would again be tested by attempting to recover from a serious injury to one of my legs.

16

$\mathcal{S}$ound of Music

Music played a major role in increasing and maintaining my desire to exercise by providing an inspirational listening environment. Allow me to explain; music adds a special dimension of enjoyment to my life and often elevates my emotions to new heights. Music allows me to get in touch with my feelings and sensitivities and can raise my spirits when I feel depressed or sorrowful. Music can also open me to experience much joy. Although there were times when I've had to turn off the music because it vividly brought back experiences or events in my life that were painful. But more often, music offers me inspiration. We all probably know how we feel when we hear music that arouses feelings of patriotism, goodness, and beauty.

When I first began working out, I saw a movie titled *Chariots of Fire*. The music from the soundtrack stirred me when I heard it, and it still does even today. The music accompanied scenes of men running as they trained to participate in the Olympics of the early 1900s. When I listened to it in the fitness room, I felt exhilarated as I exercised.

This was soon followed by another soundtrack from a movie about a boxer. This was also inspirational and gave me the desire to push beyond what I'd thought my limits were. I would feel energized to achieve higher levels of fitness and endurance. For me, music can be symbolic of efforts associated with struggles and sacrifice to achieve success and health. Inspiration can also be experienced during this struggle, whether it's physical or mental. It was important for me to struggle against negative thoughts about never reaching my goal. Overcoming these thoughts improved my self-confidence and helped me learn about my capabilities. In conversations with others regarding the importance of music, many felt it's an important stimulus. One of the attendants at the gym informed me he taped the music from the soundtrack of certain movies and played them while he worked out.

While acting as a stimulus, music tends to divert my thoughts away from discomfort. When I was writing my PhD dissertation, I discovered that music inspired me to concentrate on the subject matter and stay with it to the finish. Music acted as a stimulus that tended to increase my level of understanding and assisted me in organizing information, doing mathematical calculations, and drawing conclusions. I felt a great deal of excitement when my writings fell into place while listening to music that was uplifting. It also tends to inspire me to exercise a bit harder.

I feel we can learn more about ourselves through working out. We may feel the principal reason for working out is to achieve a high level of fitness and good health. While this should be an important objective, there are others that are as important. For me, working out cleans my system in a holistic way. It purges disturbing thoughts from my mind. It also awakens both my body and mind and allows for new information not encumbered by disagreeable experiences. There can also be a feeling of optimism that accompanies a workout. While these may be fleeting, they can help face life's challenges and successes refreshed.

17

$\mathcal{S}$oreness and Stretching

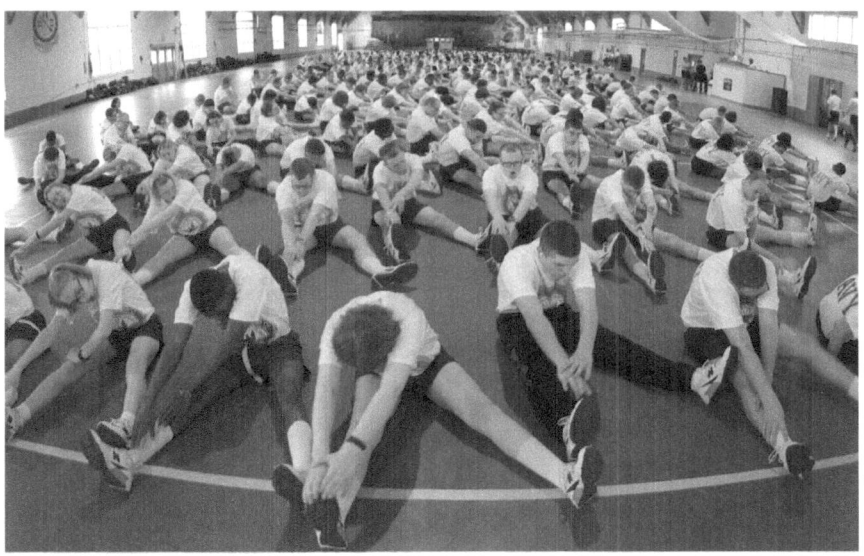

For me, an important part of exercise is stretching before and after my routine. I learned from experience with pulled muscles, sore tendons, a stiff neck, and a sore back that stretching is very important, if not absolutely necessary. My preference is to recline on a mat and stretch my whole body, part by part, before and after exercising. Most fitness centers have diagrams posted on walls displaying the various stretches one should perform. For me, stretching involves sitting on a mat, crossing my legs, and leaning forward without bending my back very much. This exercise stretches both my back and legs. Other exercises include lying on my back extending one leg straight upward and over my other leg and pulling backward on each leg with my arms. This stretches the muscle in the back of the leg (hamstring). Siting up and extending my legs outward in a V shape and leaning forward over each leg with my arms extended to touch my toes stretches my back as well as legs and arms. Sitting with my legs crossed and pushing upward with my hand on my chin stretches my neck; gently pushing my head from one side to the other also stretches my neck. I also stand and stretch my calves and Achilles heels by leaning against a wall and apply stretching pressure first on the calf of each leg and the heel and holding each of the stretching exercises for about thirty seconds. Varying this stretching routine from time to time is my basic pattern and I find it effective. If I closely follow the routine, I experience fewer strains or muscle pains. There are numerous websites that demonstrate stretching exercises for various parts of the body and I suggest viewing them to find the most appropriate ones that fit your needs.

Recently I developed a soreness at the base of both my left and right thumbs. This soreness came to my attention about a year ago and has persisted ever since. I had been using a wrist and thumb support to keep my thumbs stable while doing any bench-pressing and arm curls with free weights. This has helped, but my thumbs continue to feel sore. I decided to temporarily stop doing bench presses and shoulder exercises, which tend to place a large amount of weight onto the thumb, and switch over to doing back exercises. I also decided to see an orthopedic doctor who specializes in sports medicine. Following the examination, the doctor confirmed my suspicions and informed me that I had arthritis in my hands, specifically the wrists. He felt it was treatable with an anti-inflammatory pain-relieving cream, and a thumb brace. It was also suggested that I should refrain doing specific exercises that caused me severe pain. I was worried that if the problem was arthritis, I wouldn't be able to continue to work out with free weights. I was partially wrong, and I decided that this condition will not prevent me from continuing my fitness program. I know fully well that I will have to compensate for this issue and use lighter weights with possibly more repetitions. I also understand that I will likely discover other areas of my body affected by arthritis. This is another challenge when dealing with advancing age and its outcomes. I am confident that I will be able to compensate for whatever ailments arise and will continue to exercise.

For me, remaining fit is very important since the results allow me to continue to live an active and full life while satisfying my desire to be fit. However, for me It is necessary to periodically take a break from exercising and allow my body to rest. This period may last for at least a week or two. When I return to exercising, I discover I didn't lose much strength and found myself refreshed.

18

$\mathcal{F}$eeding the Body

Many may feel as I do, that eating is a favorite activity whether I'm hungry or not—in particular, crunchy chips that are strategically placed in food stores so that I would literally walk into them, if I wasn't paying attention. Even after seeing them on shelves, I would ponder if a new chip might have been added to the list of munchies that might contain little or no fat and cholesterol. My fantasy was, and still is to find such products and invariably seek for this elusive chip while shopping. Since never able to find it, I end up purchasing something that may satisfy my urge but has very little nutritional value and does contain some fat and cholesterol.

It's always a struggle when I food shop since I concentrate on selecting items that are seemingly healthy to eat. I discovered that after drinking skim milk for a while, not only does it taste fine, but lately when I drink 1 or even 2 percent milk, they taste too rich. Other foods I try to avoid, but not entirely, are red meat, butter, ice cream, cheese, and sometimes cake or pie. I do eat low-fat items, such as wheat breads, poultry, fish, low-fat soups, margarine, yogurt, eggs without the yolk, lots of vegetables and fruits, and of course skim milk. Much to my displeasure, I occasionally will experience a feeding frenzy and attempt to eat everything that's in the refrigerator or the kitchen cabinet. When my frenzy is satisfied, I feel guilty and lay off eating any fatty foods. When the frenzy strikes again, I try to focus on eating more fruit since this has the effect of satisfying my appetite.

Working out regularly helps to improve my eating habits. My conscience keeps reminding me that since I'm spending a great deal of time, money, and effort doing something significant to improve my health and state of mind, why ruin it by eating foods that will counteract all that good enterprise? I decided to supplement good eating habits with some vitamins. I try to take a daily multivitamin along with vitamins C and D and folic acid. There has been much press about the benefits of these vitamins, such as the possible prevention of osteoporosis as well as cancer in older citizens. Green tea is also suggested to prevent cancer in those who may be susceptible to the disease. This tea may contain polyphenols that hopefully tend to reduce free radicals. Please notice that I use the word *hopefully*! We all realize that advertising helps sell products, and whether they are beneficial appears to be debatable. It's always a person's choice on whether to use these products.

19

*A*erobic Exercise

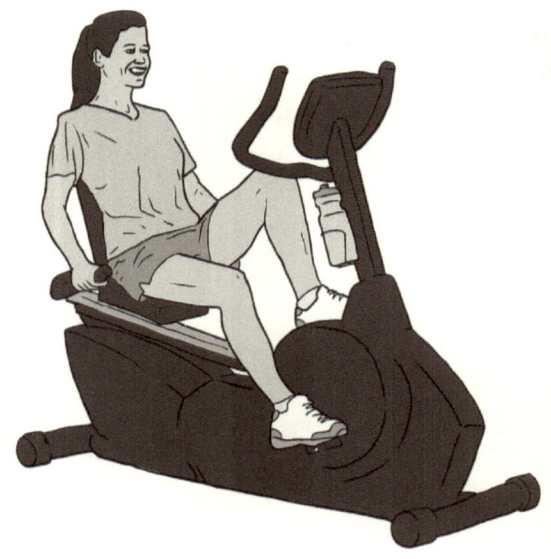

Stationary Bicycling

In time, I did find an alternative to jogging. In most gyms, there are stationary bikes that I might use for an aerobic workout or when the outside weather is nasty. While it wasn't among my favorite methods of exercise, riding on a bike for about thirty to forty-five-minutes results in achieving a good workout. It wasn't until I was living in Atlanta and exercising in a gym that I discovered an assortment of mechanical and electrical contraptions that provided excellent workouts. There were various step machines, stationary bikes, and also exercise classes available. I first tried the stationary bikes that could be programmed for numerous objectives and one's capability. As I increased my aerobic ability and eventually became bored with the bike, I switched to exercising on a step machine. I would stand and step up and down on pedals at various speeds and increase or decrease the resistance. The effect was different then exercising on the bike. As you are aware, the step machine simulates climbing stairs. Adjustments on the machine required me to step faster or slower depending on my objective. My overall goal is to be able to step or climb faster and longer over time. This exercise has some of the same cardiovascular effects as jogging. I can feel what's going on with my ability to sustain various speeds. Listening to music while I exercise tends to inspires me to push myself to acquire a high degree of aerobic ability.

Another exercise I found challenging and effective is participating in aerobic classes. The instructor stands at the front of the class and gives instructions while performing a routine that may include stepping up and down quickly and gracefully on small platforms. All this takes place to the sound of music. This routine is effective in increasing the heart rate, thereby improving the cardiovascular system. A whole routine can last up to an hour, including warm-up and cool-down phases. I found this to be similar to dancing, even though it's not necessary to have a partner. Since it is a class with others, all may enjoy doing the exercise together. Once I had memorized the steps I was able to develop a more graceful routine. As I progressed, there were instances when I felt my movements were as fluid and elegant as a dancer's.

20

Struggling with Disability

W hile working out may not be beneficial for everyone, It's difficult to think of anyone who wouldn't gain some degree of fitness. A very good friend of mine, who is partially disabled, informed me about how those who are injured view exercising. He explained that the disabled are not necessarily narcissistically directed to working out as many of us can be. However, those who are physically impaired may crave exercise on a regular basis and understand that it's essential for a reasonably healthy and active life. They are simply trying to regain a portion of what they had before the accident that struck them down. The following are several anecdotes about people I became acquainted with who struggled to overcome physical handicaps:

One of my close friends was injured one evening when he fell getting onto his houseboat. He fractured a portion of his spinal cord that left him partly paralyzed from the waist down. This accident nearly ended his life since he fell into the water and nearly drowned. Instead, he drifted helplessly into shore, where he was found the following morning by a fisherman. After an operation and months of recuperating, he could move around with the help of two walking canes. The process of rehabilitation involved working out regularly to increase mobility in his legs. Without working out, he felt he would not be able to walk at all.

When I exercised with him, I observed his routine. He spent at least an hour exercising; first on a rowing machine, and then moved from one exercise machine to another, working on his chest, arms, and back. He didn't use his cane in the gym. Sometimes he would prop himself against a wall or a machine to perform an exercise. Even though he would become discouraged, exercising helped reduce his pain. He found inspiration to continue exercising from a story told to him by an acquaintance. This story went as follows:

One day while in the gym, he spied a heavy-set man in his thirties shuffling around with obvious pain from one exercise machine to another. He concluded that this person suffered from a serious spinal cord injury, possibly similar to his own. He decided to confirm his suspicions by asking the man if this was the case. First, he revealed to this man his own tragic accident, which resulted in a nasty spinal cord injury, requiring a vertebrate fusion operation, several months recuperating in a hospital, and now finding himself struggling in the gym to improve his situation. The other man responded by telling him that he was sitting in his car in New Orleans waiting for a traffic light to turn green when a man came up out of nowhere, shoved a gun in his face, and demanded his wallet. As he reached around to retrieve it, the man shot him in the back, leaving him a paraplegic. Months later sitting in his apartment in a wheelchair, watching TV and thinking his life was over, he said to himself, "No it isn't!" I'm going to walk again even if the doctors told me it would be impossible. He then described how he wheeled himself to a door, pulled himself up out of the chair, and tried to walk. Even though he immediately fell, he kept trying. He would take a few steps and then would collapse. After a few months, his knees and elbows showed scabs from falling, but he could walk a few hundred feet. When he went outside, he would wear heavy gloves on his hands and would wrap his knees in towels. Each day he would walk a little farther. Today he still struggles, but he can walk and is attempting to live a normal life.

He then described a woman whose name is Jean who routinely came to the gym to exercise. She had twinkling eyes and a beautiful smile that radiated to all those she encountered. Jean was seventy-two, and she was paralyzed from the effects of polio and lived with pain. Her method of getting from place to place was by navigating a motorized wheelchair which she handled expertly. Jean contracted polio when she was sixteen years old. Prior to polio, she had suffered from rheumatic fever and was confined to her bed for almost six months. As she explained, years ago it was common for people to recover from illnesses in bed for a long time with very little exercise. Not so today!

Jean struggled practically her entire life with the debilitating effects of polio. During the early years of her battle, she was cared for by Christian Scientists. They would not allow her to use a wheelchair but instead required her to walk with crutches. This proved to be therapeutic and soon she could move about fairly confidently, although it left her shaking from overexertion.

In the 1980s, Jean was being cared for by a doctor who didn't recommend any kind of physical therapy and was even neutral when she informed him that she was going to undertake an exercise program at the university gym. She felt he was from the old school of "do nothing except rest when you have pain."

Eventually, she found another doctor who encouraged her to exercise. This was a doctor who felt exercise was beneficial to handicapped people. Through time, Jean developed an exercise program that served her well. It seemed to remove the constant aching and restored her sense of well-being, if not her strength. Jean's exercise program was simple enough. She walks for about ten or twelve minutes using leg braces and crutches. She then removes the braces, puts on her sneakers, and with assistance from a trainer sits on an Air-dyne stationary bike. Her feet are strapped to the pedals, and as she moves her arms back and forth on the handlebars, the pedals also move propelling her legs in an up-and-down motion. She does this peddling for about ten or twelve minutes, which amounts to one mile. After finishing with the bike routine, she does stretching exercises for about fifteen minutes, again with trainer assistance. She performs this entire routine three times a week. The stretching she can do unassisted, and she performs it every day. In addition to restoring her sense of well-being, these exercises have given her a sense of superiority, which she concludes is basically unearned and a touch unreal. On the other hand, if she fails to do this routine, she feels like a moral degenerate and is punished by ensuing pain. Jean believes her exercising not only improves her ability to cope with the situation, but also feels much better having completed it. Both joy and hope embrace her as she struggles daily to survive. She is a role model for others, as well as for me. I often think about her when dealing with my own physical issues, especially the most recent one which I will describe later in the book.

While viewing the winter Olympics, I discovered that Peggy Fleming, the very popular gold medal winner in figure skating, exercises regularly as therapy for undergoing surgery for breast cancer. Many other women have followed her example and found success.

As they have for me, perhaps these anecdotes may serve as inspiration to those who struggle to overcome physical handicaps.

21

Forward to 2015

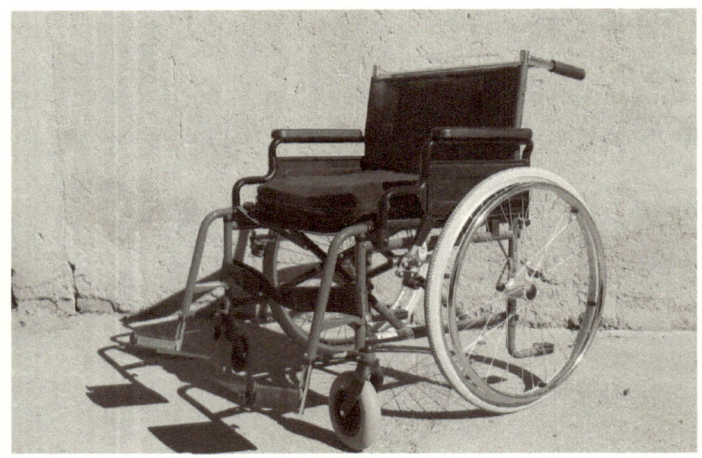

Wheelchair

In 1999, I purchased a country house near Berkeley Springs in West Virginia. The area is moderately forested and inhabited by abundant wildlife, especially deer. While there, we enjoy swimming in the western part of the Potomac River, where it's narrow and fairly shallow. Walking in wooded areas and viewing abundant plant and wildlife, including trees and birds is also enjoyable.

All was going well until the spring of 2015 when my wife and I both suffered serious accidents. While descending the circular stairway from the upper floor to the lower level, she fell and severely broke her left ankle. I heard her scream and rushed to her side. Seeing and hearing the pain she was in, I called for an ambulance to rush her to a hospital that was located in Winchester, Virginia. Over a period of several days, I visited while she was recuperating from two operations on four broken bones in her ankle.

Three days later at my house, I encountered a nest of wasps on the first floor deck. While spraying them with wasp deterrent, I slipped on the residue and fell. I twisted my leg in such a way that my right knee felt severely injured. As I lay on the deck, I tried but could not stand as my leg was incapable of holding my weight. I was also in a great deal of pain. Realizing I required medical help, I remembered the phone was just inside the deck door sitting on a table. I began pushing myself backward on the deck and eventually made it through the sliding door into the first floor. To get to the phone, I pushed the table until the phone fell on the floor. I picked it up and called the emergency number for assistance to transport me to a hospital. While I sat on the floor, I was breathing hard and tried to control my anxiety. I felt confused about what happened to me. It wasn't long before an ambulance arrived and while being transported to a hospital the attendant kept me busy by asking questions about all sorts of things. I later discovered this was a strategy to keep me from fainting. I found it reassuring to be gently spoken to. I kept thinking about how foolish it was to attempt getting rid of the wasps. I recalled being both angry and fearful that they appeared to be invading my space. They were actually building a nest for themselves and paying me no attention. I feel I should have done the same.

At the hospital in Martinsburg, West Virginia. I was given a medical examination, and it was determined that I had severed the main ligament in my right knee and required an operation. This was to be the first major operation I would experience in my life. Following the operation, and an initial recovery of a few days, arrangements were made to transport me to Ingleside facility in Washington, DC, to begin recovery and receive physical therapy. In addition, it was determined that my wife would also convalesce at

Ingleside. Strange as it may sound, it appeared that our accidents, the assistance and medical attention we both received occurred at the same place and nearly the same time.

Ingleside provided us with our own private rooms and the opportunity to receive therapy to begin the healing process. I envisioned it would take a long time to regain adequate motion in my right leg. I needed to wear a leg brace that encased the entire leg from my crotch to my ankle. After arriving and settling into my room, I realized we both had gone through a most difficult time, and more was certain to follow. That first evening, I began to weep and did so for quite a while. When I finally stopped, I prayed for the strength to see us through the difficult period ahead.

The resident fitness instructors who supervised therapy appeared to be well trained. Each day an instructor would arrive at my room to escort me to the fitness area. On our way there, she would take me outside the building and we would walk where retired people lived in row houses or apartments. I enjoyed talking to those who were sitting outside reading. In time, I became friendly with several and looked forward to seeing and talking with them. After greeting them all, I would enter the building where the fitness area was located. I spent about an hour doing various rudimentary exercises for my leg. At first, it was frustrating to only be able to perform simple exercises. I realized it would take a long time before I would be as agile and strong when before my accident, if that was even possible.

The days appeared to drag by, and it appeared the exercises were not helping me improve. In actuality, I was improving little by little even though it was hardly noticeable. I remembered reading that making improvements in strength do not necessarily happen at a constant rate and my responses seemed to bear this out. After a while, I began experiencing improvement in both the strength of my leg and its mobility. For example, there were periods when I could remove the leg brace and walk without it. This had a positive impact on my psyche, and I was beginning to believe I may walk normally again.

Over a period of about a month, my knee began to feel much

better but not completely healed. I had to continue wearing the leg brace. It eventually became clear to the staff director that the time arrived for me to return home and seek local rehabilitation. In addition, my health insurance was running out for this level of care. Feeling a bit nervous about leaving, I pulled the proverbial ripcord and left by cab. During the trip home, I had some opposing feelings during that trip home; some good and some fearful.

Even though my leg is still recovering, I now make it a priority to walk quickly while on vacation, even in places I never visited before. This offers the opportunity to fully experience the local environment. Jogging will have to wait until I'm fully recovered.

22

$\mathcal{R}$eturning Home

Returning home was not easy since I had to become accustomed to not being cared for. My wife had returned earlier, but I couldn't rely on her assistance and had to gingerly use a walker to get around. Fortunately, her daughter stayed with us and was helpful in preparing meals and assisting in any way she could. It finally came time for her to return to her apartment. We both needed to fend for ourselves and I was still reliant on my leg brace during the day. We are very appreciative of neighbors who prepared meals for us.

After several weeks and visits to my doctor, it was concluded I could remove the leg brace. This was good news since I could begin exercising at home and also assist my wife. No longer did I have to remain indoors. I could take walks outside, first with the brace on and then finally without it. It was a major event when I finally removed the brace for the last time. At first, I felt a bit vulnerable. However, it didn't take long to celebrate its disappearance from my life. For a short time, I stored it in the basement and then finally discarded it. When walking outside, I enjoyed meeting neighbors and hearing local news. Since I am an outside type of person, I was delighted to once again being back in the environment.

A beautiful park is near the house, and I could walk to it and enjoy the vegetation and a fast-flowing creek. Having been deprived from being outside for some time, I was overjoyed to begin immersing myself back into nature. As a geologist, it has been and still is very important to view and reflect on forms and structures of our planet. Challenging myself to interpret what I viewed in the neighborhood helped keep my mind active. Also, being a naturalist and seeing birds, squirrels, and people's pets was also a treat.

I started doing physical exercises at home since I wasn't prepared to drive to the neighborhood fitness center. The exercises I performed were fairly basic. Since it had been nearly six months without doing aerobic exercises, I began by sitting on a chair while moving my arms in various directions to increase my respiration. This exercise gave me the desired aerobic result. As time went by, I increased the time and I began taking walks in the neighborhood. These walks began slowly and increased in distance over time. It felt good to once again to be able to see the geological structures in the immediate area.

One day when I was out in the neighborhood, I met a neighbor who in the past experienced a leg injury similar to my own. Even though he is younger than me, I felt he clearly understood what I was going through. While we were talking, I told him about problems with my car battery and also lighting the ceramic plates in our fireplace. Since he was a mechanical engineer, I thought he might provide me with possible solutions. After listening, he offered to fix these issues. It didn't take me long to gladly accept his offer. He fixed the battery by cleaning the connections that had become corroded. He had a tool that was specially designed for tackling the problem. He then removed and cleaned the ceramic plates in the fireplace, which took a considerable amount of time. He positioned the plates back in the holder and the fireplace could be ignited. After quite a few years it was now useable and we looked forward to its orange color and warmth on cold evenings. I was thankful for his assistance and felt fortunate to have him as not only a neighbor but also a friend.

During my time being sequestered, there were other instances when I felt fortunate. Maintaining friendships is very important and especially when you're having trouble just getting around. Re-establishing my relationship with this neighbor turned out to be very worthwhile and I hope he felt the same. This also occurred between other neighbors and my wife. Even though they are also my friends, they have known my wife for years and in some respects, you might say they all grew older and wiser together.

I began sharing with my children and close friends some of the difficult challenges we faced and felt it was especially helpful to talk about it. Most of the time I tend to hold personal information close to the chest. The reasons for doing so is mostly attributed to feeling shy, embarrassed, and possibly being thought of as stupid.

Recently I was on the phone talking to a friend in Virginia and heard about his weakening health. We are the same age and have been friends since we were eighteen years old. I have another friend living nearby who attended the same high school on Staten Island and played football with me. During my time being sequestered, I would communicate with them both, and found this helpful and at times hilarious. Humor always seemed to be common when I spoke to each of them and this kept my mind off any troubles. I came to realize I wasn't the only person dealing with a difficult situation. Many people don't have close friends for this long, and I am truly grateful.

$\mathcal{B}$eginning Again

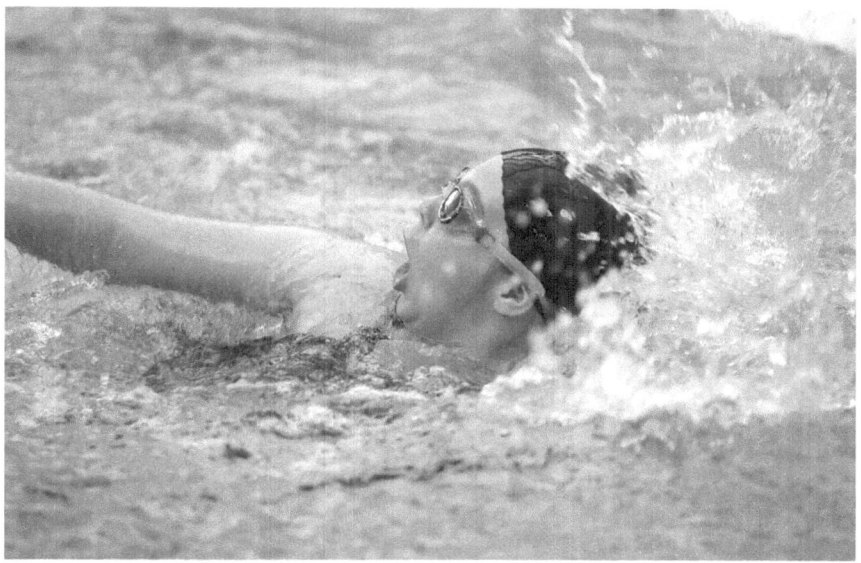

Swimming Pool

While it seemed it took forever, I felt I could finally begin exercising in earnest. I decided to try swimming at a nearby High School pool. Even though the school is less than two miles from our door step, I had never swum in the pool. In fact, I wasn't even aware of its existence until a neighbor told me about it. It's an indoor Olympic-size pool with twelve lanes, including all the accessories for changing clothes, showers, and lockers. There is also a smaller pool for both adults and children. The pool and facilities are available at no cost to DC residents anytime during the day and early evening. Even though I didn't feel ready to return to the fitness center, I did feel prepared to swim to get myself back in shape.

I began by swimming in the lane reserved for slow swimmers. In the beginning, I would swim for about fifteen minutes before feeling tired and needing to stop. I felt discouraged that I was so out of condition I couldn't swim longer. I recall last summer when we were on vacation at my wife's family vacation home in Pennsylvania, I could swim for only a short time even while my legs were often touching the lake bottom. Even so, I kept it up and did achieve some benefit along with gaining confidence about swimming for exercise.

Swimming at this local pool has become very important to regain being fit again. I try to swim at least two to three days a week. Lately I swim for forty-five minutes without resting. Even when I was healthy and without an injury, I can't recall when I would swim continuously for that long. Recently, I swam for a full fifty minutes—the longest time yet! While swimming, my breathing is steady and I'm feeling strong. I appreciate why others feel this is one of the best exercises to increase one's strength, stamina, and overall health. I am now a firm supporter of that opinion.

I often observe others in lanes designated for those who swim fast and I'm envious. Even so, I realize that I'm gradually improving both my speed and endurance. While swimming, I have many different thoughts. Even though they're not focused on anything specific, I find them stimulating. I enjoy looking beneath the water's surface and recall vacations when I would watch various types of fish swimming near and around me. I also observe how others move their legs in the water, and if it seems reasonable, I try to copy them. Increases in my ability takes time, and I'm beginning to understand it's a slow process. It has taken me nearly six months to achieve what I now can perform. It will likely take several more months to achieve my next goal of swimming for one hour or more without resting.

Even though at this time I hadn't returned to the nearby fitness facility to exercise, I felt it wouldn't be much longer. Swimming provides many benefits for my condition that include strengthening my limbs, aerobic conditioning, and weight control. Additionally, the urge to swim becomes stronger each time I go. I've become a steady user of this facility and I appreciate my ability each time I go. Aside from these benefits, I have become attached to the process as never before. This has not only been therapy for my knee, but it's reason to enjoy living again. It involves a process that includes planning, arriving at the pool, dressing to swim, and finally immersing myself in the pool. After completing my swim, relaxing in the whirlpool brings comfort to my body. Following getting dressed and returning to the world, whether warm or cold outside, I feel refreshed and prepared to face whatever awaits me in life.

24

$\mathcal{R}$eturn to the Fitness Center

It finally came time to return to exercise at the nearby fitness facility. This was my conclusion based on how I felt both physically and mentally. Even so, I felt wary about this venture. When I arrived, the staff greeted me warmly. They had been informed of what happened to both myself and my wife. It felt good to be among those who support our desire to be healthy and fit again. Much to my delight, they were knowledgeable about dealing with those who had suffered injuries like ours. I decided to begin exercising by walking on the treadmill. This worked out well since I could vary its speed by going slow at first and steadily increase it over time. I also could vary the time spent on the treadmill. I started walking for about twenty minutes at a slow speed. Overtime, I began increasing both the time and eventually the speed. I could walk for about thirty minutes or more while periodically increasing the speed. I also began working out on the exercise machines and it was slow going at first.

There are different machines for different parts of the body. I focused on exercising both my legs since I wanted them to be as strong as possible. I would use equipment where I would push various amounts of weight upward from a lying position, first using both legs, then just one leg along with varying the amount of weight. I initially discovered that my left leg is stronger than the injured one. Though recently, the injured leg has grown much stronger and can press nearly the same amount of weight as the other one. This is a vast improvement in strength, which pleases me. I owe this improvement to being consistent in doing the exercises.

To vary my routine, I continue to swim. I now focus on swimming at the pool and exercising at the fitness center. For me, this feels like the perfect combination for becoming healthy and fit again. The resident instructors agree this was a good routine which makes me feel I'm doing the right things for myself. Swimming is perfect for all-around fitness that includes strengthening the legs and upper body while providing anaerobic benefits. Exercising at the facility has similar effects, but focuses more on building the musculature of legs and upper body. As I did earlier, I include stretching my body before and following weight training. This helps to relieve any stiffness and soreness in my muscles prior and following exercising.

While both types of exercise provide some similar benefits, there are important differences. Being in a large open area where people are swimming can be enjoyable since it may remind us of enjoyable vacations. It also provides opportunities to observe others that invoke memories of swimming with friends and family members. The pool area may include a whirlpool where one can sit, stretch, and enjoy the warm, turbulent water massaging the body. This has the effect of loosening the musculature and improving circulation. It's similar to receiving a massage from a masseur. An important issue may include not having the ability to swim. Even so, walking in shallow water is beneficial since resistance of the water requires using leg muscles and provides aerobic conditioning. I have watched others doing this exercise and I assume for the same reason. I also enjoy doing it when I finish swimming. I would highly recommend getting in the water when and if you can.

At the fitness center, I focus on exercising various parts of my body. As opposed to swimming, there can be more than just one exercise to obtain benefits. As described earlier, each exercise machine is designed to have an effect on a part or possibly several parts of the body. For example, there are machines for exercising upper leg musculature, biceps, abdominal and back muscles.

To improve cardiovascular systems, there are classes in aerobic exercise that are available most days, as well as treadmills and step machines. They are all effective. Along with expert advice from trainers, participants can decide for themselves which kind of aerobic and weight training is best depending upon their availability. For me, the combination of both swimming at the pool and exercising at the fitness center is ideal.

25

Swimming and Exercise

I discovered that varying the kinds of exercises provide the best results. As I wrote earlier, I currently swim at the pool two to three days a week and exercise in the fitness center about the same amount of time. I vary this routine to keep from becoming bored, and it appears to work well. I thereby gain aerobic benefits as well as strengthening my body. It has taken me awhile to adjust to this routine; now I am thankful I can do so successfully. If one is healing or recuperating from an injury or illness, it's best to have patience and go slow. While doing this can be frustrating, it's important not to reinjure a limb or prevent the process of healing. Each of us may differ in how we respond to exercise. That's why it's important to obtain advice from a medical doctor or health practitioner before going forward with physical activity following an injury. The time I spent recuperating from knee surgery was about three to four weeks before I could begin exercising. I took it slow and easy until I completed going to the rehabilitation center at the Washington Hospital Center.

For me, swimming is a bit more enjoyable than exercising with weights. While both are important, the surrounding environment while swimming is enjoyable to experience. Especially watching the activity around the pool and viewing different swimming styles people use. I recall my own pleasure swimming in various places during my life, especially as both a young child and teenager.

For example, as a child, swimming at Hampton Ponds near Holyoke was always enjoyable. Living on Staten Island I would swim at the city pool, where I worked part-time selling snacks. Over the past several years, swimming with my wife at a lake in Pennsylvania is always enjoyable; even in the fall of 2015 when we were recuperating from leg injuries. We would sit on the lawn by the lake and cautiously walk holding hands into the water and begin swimming. Being a much better swimmer then me, she would swim quickly out from shore, and I would follow more slowly. Sometimes we would swim laps within a line of floats. I would often complete swimming sooner since I would tire. When she finished swimming, I would walk up and help her out of the water by holding her hand. I felt that others sitting on the grassy area might think how nice it was that I would go down and assist her. I wondered what they might have thought when seeing this expression of caring for each other. We will swim there again in upcoming weeks and future summers. If I have the nerve, I may ask someone on the beach what they thought about when they saw us walking hand in hand out of the water. Is it possible this might make a difference in someone's life?

To digress a bit, there are numerous examples of caring and reaching out to assist one another in moments of need. After all, we are human, and acts of kindness, love, and offering assistance are part of our hallmark. I began wondering about these expressions. Do they only apply to us?

I recently read about the killing of elephants in Africa for their tusks which in certain countries are in great demand and very expensive. It's also been reported that the behavior of elephants following the death of another appears to resemble acts of grieving; not very different from our own when losing a family member or a close one. Elephants commonly will remain near one of their own for several days and exhibit feelings of tenderness or grief by touching or rubbing it with their trunk before moving on. This behavior is not restricted to only elephants. Other wildlife expresses some sort of emotion after one of their kind dies, including birds. They may behave erratically when one of their young dies or becomes lost. Dogs may also show remorse by howling or lying still when they lose one of their pups or even their master. While the behavior of animals may be both similar and different from our own, we should be aware that life, whatever it may look like, may share similar responses to situations as our own.

Recently I was visiting the Washington Zoo and watched several orangutans at the top of a tall structure holding onto ropes that extended to another nearby structure about one hundred feet away. While the crowd below was watching, they in turn were looking at the crowd. Then, with one following the other, they swung themselves forward on the ropes, moving to the a nearby structure. It appeared they wanted the crowd below to watch them swing themselves across. It was beautiful to witness their ability to move so gracefully. I wished I could move as gracefully as they did. I then recalled there are entertainers in the circus who can be nearly as graceful on a high wire.

26

ℒearning Who I Am

A
s being a geologist and an oceanographer, staying fit is important if I wanted to remain physically active in these careers. Seeking to identify geologic features in the field may require heavy-duty walking, climbing, and arm strength. The purpose is to collect samples of sediment or rock and when possible, fossils. Collecting requires adequate strength to dig into outcrops and remove samples. In some instances, these outcrops are difficult to reach and require climbing steep slopes. I found this to be the case on numerous occasions. There were times when I had to rely on my ability to climb to areas where I needed to take samples of both sediment and fossils. Also, as an oceanographer, being able to swim in areas where strong currents and waves exist is important and may be necessary. I feel my emphasis on being fit prepared me to deal with physical challenges that often confront earth scientists. Later in my life, I found that I would be challenged even again.

When I was employed at the Smithsonian Institution, the senior geologist I worked for asked me to accompany him on a geologic expedition to Colorado and Wyoming. The purpose was to collect fossils and map a specific area. My family accompanied me on this trip. While hiking through an area, I decided to take my 3-year old daughter and walk through a dense forested area to eventually view the landscape. After about an hour and having my daughter on my shoulders, I began to realize we were lost. This frightened me. My daughter appeared to feel my concern and asked me,

"Are we lost, Daddy?" After reassuring her that we were not lost, I remembered to focus on controlling my breathing and think positively about having the patience to find our way back to the main path. It wasn't long before I found the path and others in the group. I feel that being in good physical condition gave me a clear presence of mind to deal with that small crisis and not panic, especially in front of my daughter.

Staying fit has helped me numerous times to complete tasks that required focus, strength and endurance. For example, assisting my mentor collect and describe fossils, especially on very hot days in the summer, tested my ability to complete whatever task was necessary. I was thankful for being in shape and able to follow his directions without difficulty. I clearly understood that physical fitness is very important for a geologist. There were instances when having the ability to climb steep slopes and excavate sediment to extract samples of both the fossils and sediment was important for later study. I learned that performing geological investigations in the field required being in decent shape, and this provided additional incentive to exercise frequently.

27

$\mathcal{R}$ecent Fitness Information

While reading a local newspaper, I came across an article about exercise and health. There was a study on exercise that reported America's couch potato lifestyle was beyond what people imagined it to be. It suggested that many people were not exercising, and many of them were not even moving. Additionally, this information suggested this was also true for those in their twenties through their forties. The researcher's goals were to determine what we must do to improve heart health and live longer. Is it necessary for a person to exercise daily, or is it okay to be a weekend warrior? Additionally, are brief, high-intensity workouts just a fad, or do they actually work? According to this science initiative, what they didn't know is what is the right dose of exercise?

The article also went on to report on a publication by an epidemiologist. This study compared workers who worked in pairs on the same shifts on double-decker buses. While breathing the same air, there was a difference in their routine. The drivers spent most of their time sitting while the conductors walked up and down the aisles selling tickets and climbed about six hundred steps each shift. In analyzing the data, it was concluded something quite significant; over a two-year period, the conductors were 50 percent less likely to suffer a heart attack than the drivers.

While this was only one study that demonstrated that exercise can be beneficial to one's health, it's a hallmark for the kind of information about results gained from exercising. Other similar studies will likely follow in the future. I can think of no one who has complained that exercise has not been beneficial to his or her life.

My own recovery and improvements from exercising, swimming and walking are many and still continue. I feel that along with my body, they have enhanced both my mind and spirit. I feel confident that facing adversity, whatever form it may take, and striving to overcome it is the best option that one can do for themselves as well as others.

28

$\mathcal{M}$y Friend's Struggle

I was recently informed by the wife of a longtime friend that he appears to be physically unstable and can no longer remain in his house. He requires medical care and supervision in a hospital or some other type of care facility. I knew he was ill and wasn't able to move around much by himself. We have been friends since we were both eighteen years old—by my count over fifty years ago. Although, even as friends we are quite different. For example, I wanted to be healthy and he didn't seem to feel that was important. The best explanation for our friendship is there was common ground between us since we both enjoyed fishing, boating, and girls! We also liked to drink beer. As with many young men, we were in competition, albeit friendly, with each other. This occasionally took the form of who was the better fisherman and who was most attractive to girls.

These are common traits among young men, and it's likely the same even now. I do admire him, and I felt he was like a brother who seemed to fill a gap in my life. Another important point; he was in the Marine Corps Reserves. With the permission of his parents, he enlisted when he turned seventeen years old. His father was a career marine with an exemplary service record and he wanted to follow in his footsteps. It wasn't long before I decided to join the Marine Corps Reserves. I was very envious of the way his uniform fit him. It was always well tailored while mine always seemed to be loose fitting. I discovered later his mother took charge of tailoring and ironing his uniform until it appeared perfect. What a break for him!

In 1968, my friend volunteered to go on active duty and serve in Vietnam. I recall that I envied his decision and wanted to volunteer myself. I was married at the time, and we had two children. I was working on my master's degree and felt it would be irresponsible of me to leave my family and go on active duty. While in Vietnam, he wrote me several letters and described what he saw and experienced, which wasn't pleasant. After completing his one-year tour of duty, he safely returned home. He was proud to have been promoted to staff sergeant. He had also lost much weight and appeared very fit. His time in the Marine Corps demanded he be in good physical condition.

Soon thereafter, he enlisted in the Navy Seabee reserves to continue his military service and earn a retirement. For his dedicated service, he continued being promoted until he could retire as a senior chief. Along with another close friend of his, I was invited to attend his retirement ceremony. It was a joyous occasion, and he was pleased we attended. His acceptance speech of retirement to the attending audience was excellent. His speech only broke a few times as emotion welled up in his voice, and this added sincerity in his farewell to the Seabees. His farewell will continue to evoke much emotion in me.

29

$\mathcal{W}$hat's Next?

To me, it's obvious that working out can help prepare us seniors, as well as others, to participate more fully in all aspects of living. Paying attention to exercising increases our opportunity to be involved in all aspects of living well into our senior years. It's also my opinion that working out not only improves the quality of our lives, which includes our physical, emotional, and possibly intellectual abilities, but may allow us to more fully enter into a spiritual existence. As we become fit and improve our health, we may find the energy and desire to explore the meaning of our lives. Working out demands concentration and dedication. Attaining spiritual fulfillment may also require the same concentration, meditation, and dedication. Exercising is a lifelong commitment. There are no quick fixes or shortcuts to become healthy and fit. This is a total life experience, and I'm convinced the benefits far outweigh the costs necessary to achieve this outcome.

Having come full circle with my desire to be fit and healthy, the road ahead looks much better than a couple of years ago. Regardless of my age, I am not the type of person to sit on my laurels and wait for something to happen. As I examine my abilities, I conclude that I want to write not only this book but others as well.

At this time in my life, I realize I will continue to work out for as long as possible to keep myself healthy. To my knowledge, there are no signposts that may caution me to refrain from this activity. We must make up our own minds about going forward to meet challenges that confront us. In doing so, we may discover much about ourselves, including limits we place in our path. I feel that moving in this manner instills self-confidence to take on new enterprises. I am not aware of anything written that suggests we should not challenge ourselves and attempt to discover who we are. I feel when we hold back from going forward, it's primarily ourselves and not something else that prevents us.

When I was a graduate student in 1970, I would jog to keep my anxiety in check. My son, who was about four years old, would try to run along with me. This lifted my spirits since I felt he wanted to be with me no matter what we did together. He would trail along with me until he ran out of breath. Often when I'd be working out, I would think about his desire to be with me. Lately I feel I could have slowed up a bit and allowed him to keep up with me. I also could have been more encouraging about his desire to be with me. I feel instilling the desire for maintaining fitness in our children will ultimately benefit them. Our impact on others may be unknown, other than to realize it may be significant.

Since my children are aware how important it's been for me to exercise, they continue to encourage me. I hope I have set myself as an example for them. To do that, I need to continue exercising in a sense for all of us. Recently, my daughter told me that after working out at a gym, she felt both exhausted but physically quite good. I hope I influenced her to exercise even though she's now in her early fifties and has three small children. While talking to her recently, she sounded proud of herself to have completed exercising. I gloated at hearing this since I was taking some credit for her focus and endurance. There are times when I feel she resembles me, especially when it comes to exercising. My son and I are also closely connected through many things, including our love of sports—especially rooting for the local professional teams. We also enjoy fishing together, especially when my boat is useable and we actually catch fish.

I also feel they appreciate I engage in activities that bring me pleasure. I often wonder if they feel drawn to do things that also provide me satisfaction. I assume most parents feel the same. There are many ways we can influence our children, and I hope what I do helps them decide on a good path of life to follow. I also hope they will not take some paths I followed where I had to spend much time making amends and corrections.

Exercising has helped me deal with unknowns in my life. Some still exist and will likely remain since much of life can be unknown. However, I feel that following a path of being healthy and able to face the future is best for both me and for those that are close. I wish to be healthy and able to be there for others when difficulties arise that cause pain and sorrow. Being able to come forward with love and caring are what I want to give to others in difficult times.

30

$\mathscr{L}$earning about Myself

A s I move forward in life, my desire to help others has become strong and difficult to ignore. When confronted with this realization, I initially felt I was too involved in other pressing endeavors. As I began to examine them, I realized they were not that important. As one who has reached an advanced age and accumulated some worthwhile experience, why not share it? That's one reason I'm writing this book. I have repeatedly asked myself, isn't it important to share our difficulties and successes with those who may gain insight into what might be useful in their lives? I'm sure most of us have felt this weight of accumulated knowledge and wished we could lighten our load. This can be achieved by sharing it with others who can apply it in their own situations.

I have often asked myself whether the sharing of information with others has been useful. As a professor for many years, I shared much information with students about my experiences associated with topics I taught. It was through this sharing that I learned more about the subject matter and hopefully the students benefitted. Additionally, it has occurred that the interests of some students coincided with my own and would lead to in-depth discussions on subjects that went beyond the scope of an assignment. I was fortunate to receive positive feedback from those who graduated from the program, and this made me feel my work was useful and appreciated. I feel this can be a part of our experience while exercising.

We can learn about benefits associated with various exercises as we continue using them in our routine. If there is an exercise that doesn't feel right for whatever reason, it may be best to discontinue using it. I have done this trial and error with different exercises. With the assistance of a trainer, I was able to identify the best routine for me, especially one that challenged the major muscle groups and resulted in me feeling good.

While I continue with exercising, other feelings and desires have begun to occupy my mind. Occasionally, I question the reasons for why I'm motivated. I realize there is no simple answer. It could be as simple as, "I really don't know." The feedback I give myself is, "That's just not good enough." I have been seeking answers to similar questions that have plagued me for a long time. I revealed much about myself in this writing, and while doing so, I have come face-to-face with myself. Unsettling as it may seem, I discovered things I was unaware of. As my story unfolded, memories came flooding back into my mind. Some were not easy to reveal and would cause me to take a pause from writing. Others were joyful and brought back pleasant memories and even tears of joy.

I've asked myself repeatedly why am I so dedicated to exercising and attempting to remain fit even after dealing with crises and disappointments. My response to this question has to do with, "Who am I?" Isn't this what we all ask ourselves time and time again? Doesn't learning who we are take a long time to discover? There are available books that have explored this question, and I will cite one that I am currently reading: *The Untethered Soul* by Michael A. Singer.

I understand that I have come to know myself better than if I never exercised. Experiencing the feelings of dedication and accomplishment, even failure, have taught me much about myself. Exercising is an adventure that never really ends. However, there continues to be events that can slow this activity or bring it to a halt. During my lifetime, injuries have caused this to occur several times. In either case, my desire to exercise continued to be active. I had to learn to be patient and allow myself to recover and regain the ability to become active again. Being patient isn't easy. If you are like me, I tend to be impatient and wish to see results quickly. I realize this may be impossible, so I had to learn about acquiring patience. I discovered that others could help me achieve this seemingly impossible state of being. Those who did, and still do, provide assistance include family members, doctors, nurses, fitness instructors, and a physical therapist.

I want to emphasize the importance of having patience when injured, and I had to learn it early on. Taking small steps and taking one's time to recover, along with supervision, is critical and the only way to go. I often felt discouraged about my progress while a part of me kept insisting I was ignoring my improvement. I tried ignoring a pesky voice that would tell me there is little hope. It appeared my mind was dwelling more on negative outcomes instead of being positive. I finally realized that along with physical rehabilitation, my mental state and outlook also needed refurbishment. In time and with every achievement, regardless of how small, I began to become mentally stronger.

As the summer of 2016 was in full swing, I felt good about my progress. Taking time to enjoy being with friends and relations. Because of my earlier knee surgery, there was little opportunity to travel. Now that I was feeling better, I wanted to be more active, especially during the arriving summer. Along with my wife, I prepared to join two friends of mine with their wives for three full days at a beautiful house in Virginia. These friends were high school chums of mine when I lived on Staten Island. We played football together on our High School team in 1954. Even though it was long ago, my memories of being with them are crystal clear. Although I may forget what I did a day or so ago, these earlier memories have stayed with me. We have kept our friendships active by routinely getting together over the past several years, especially in having dinner with our wives.

We all were looking forward to spending a few days together in a fantastic house located in a mountain setting in Virginia. We planned to do much while being together. While I wouldn't be swimming or going to a gym, we planned to do much walking in the area. I did continue to exercise not only my leg but as much of myself as possible.

This part of Virginia is not only scenic, but it also has an interesting geological history. Being a geologist, I wish to provide the reader with a snapshot of this history. The mountain we were on is part of a system that is approximately three hundred million years old. The mountains at that time were possibly twenty thousand feet high, whereas currently their elevation is about three thousand feet. The North Atlantic plate, of which the East Coast was a part, collided with the European plate and formed that early mountain range, which currently is significantly smaller. Erosion over millions of years is responsible for its much-smaller presence on the East Coast. Erosion is still active and studies suggest it is occurring at a rate of two to three inches per year. This doesn't sound like a lot, but over millions of years, it is significant.

Prior to going to Virginia, my wife and I planned to travel to our getaway house in West Virginia to spend several days. While there and if weather permitted, we would swim in the Potomac River. As usual, swimming is always a great exercise for our injuries. We have swum there many times, even when the current has been swift. My wife enjoys swimming across the river to the opposite bank, while I stay on the near side swimming laps parallel to the shore. The water tends to be quite clear and fairly shallow, and often we can see small fish swimming and jumping out of the water. While some people from a nearby campground also swim there, much of the time we are the only ones. The views of the river both upstream and downstream are quite striking. Many trees growing close to its banks tend to bend down close to the water. Some have uprooted and fallen into the river creating habitats for fish. There are no houses visible, only trees and other vegetation. Occasionally, a train can be heard and seen passing over the river on a bridge. There are trailers nearby where the owners come to stay for several days, although their presence doesn't diminish the scenic setting. After purchasing the house, I was delighted there was this place nearby to swim. The environment was suitable since I enjoy a more rustic setting for swimming and especially since its never crowded.

In addition to swimming, and provided it's not raining, it's a pleasure to walk within open fields and a heavily wooded area that includes an association of homes as well as near my house. Most of the area is hilly since it's a part of the foothills of the Appalachian Mountains. Traffic in the area is non-existent, especially at night. When standing or sitting on the deck of my house in late evening, only headlights can occasionally be seen on the road. Cars are more frequently seen or heard when residents are traveling to and from work.

You might think finding a gym or fitness center would be difficult while being distant from a population center. About nine miles west is a town called Berkeley Springs and is known for the spring water that flows to the surface from an underground source. Residents feel this water may have health benefits to those who drink it. Berkeley Springs is also the county seat for Berkeley County and is a thriving community that contains stores, shops, service stations, schools, restaurants, and a fitness center. I have been using this facility for several years and especially lately to strengthen my leg. When I'm in West Virginia, there is no excuse to not exercise. As I mentioned earlier, there is a large demand for places to exercise and West Virginia is no exception. The attendance at the fitness center is fairly high. What also makes this center attractive is the presence of a cadre of professionals who are medically trained to assist in determining what method of exercise is appropriate for the attendees. Since I only take advantage of this facility when I am at my house, I follow the routine I would use if I were in DC.

This year I went swimming in the river for the first time in nearly two years. The current was swift, but I did my best to keep swimming upstream. If I swam with the current, I would find myself downstream in no time. Periodically, I had to touch bottom with my feet and give myself a push to keep on the surface. It wasn't optimal, but I did get a pretty good workout using this method.

When we travel to Laport, PA in the summer to stay at my wife's family house, there is a fitness center nearby where I can exercise. It appears that wherever I travel to there are always places to exercise.

31

The Team

As mentioned in the previous chapter, I received a message from a high school classmate of mine that he wanted me along with another classmate of ours, including wives, to get together for several days. This would take place at the house of his daughter and son-in-law in the mountains of Virginia. This was a terrific opportunity for us to finally be together since we played football on our high school team in 1952. I leaped at the chance and we all met at the house in Virginia in June 2016.

Soon after we all were together, memories of attending school and playing football together came back in a rush. I couldn't recall each and every game we played in, but I remembered several times when I caught a pass thrown to me by the quarterback. I also remembered several plays my friends were involved in-especially when one of them tackled a runner from the other team in his own backfield for a loss of several yards. I'm not sure I would have recalled our playing football together unless we were together during those several days.

Except for one friend who lives close by in Virginia, I had not been in frequent touch with my other friend. Our reunion has changed that and we all have found reasons to contact one another more frequently. In fact, my more distant friend sent us articles about both subjects and trips we might be interested in. I recently received from one of them a description of our get-together, along with a photo he intends to send to the high school we attended. He hopes the administration will publish it in their school paper.

I feel that continuing to be in touch with one another will strengthen the bonds between us. In my mind, friendships are very important and deserve to be continually refreshed by sharing information about what's happening in each of our lives. Hopefully this will keep our friendships active and demonstrate we truly care for one another. I also feel this sharing will help us appreciate that even though our lives may be complex and somewhat erratic, we will all remain close friends. Our families who witness this caring and appreciation we have for one another may help them understand the importance of keeping in touch with their friends.

Along with our wives, we spent time conversing about our lives, as well as our children's. It was startling to hear some of their life's stories. We all seemed to have much experience in dealing with life's demands, and that included both rewards and setbacks. I talked about the injury to my leg and how it curtailed many of my activities. I heard accounts from each of them about finding their own pathways in life. For all of us, some paths were blind alleys, whereas others brought us to where we currently are. As I described mine, I felt tears well up in my eyes. This display of emotional feelings seemed fine while I was among my oldest of friends. They in turn not only showed deep interest but also added their own paths to this potpourri. We spent considerable time exchanging stories, which also included experiences from the women. Being together provided the opportunity to experience and know one another as older adults. Although we missed sharing many important events we each had, it didn't appear to hinder us from effectively communicating with one another.

Over the past few years, I spent more time with my friend who lives in Virginia than with the one who is distant from us both. However, my connection with him quickly strengthened as we were all together. When our time finally ended, we went our separate ways heading home. I feel we will take the opportunity to meet again and further strengthen the bond that brought us together in the first place. I am quite sure we will remain good friends for the time that remains for each of us, and that is a most welcome gift.

32

$\mathcal{S}$haring the Experience

An important part of being fit is being able to convince others about the importance of fitness in their lives. My children are busy with work, their own children, and running a household. With her husband and three young ones, my daughter is very busy attending to their needs. For quite a while when they were very small, she didn't have time to exercise. Taking care of her children and being available to her husband occupied all her time. As I wrote earlier, she's been able to return to a gym and exercise. We have communicated about the importance of exercising and how it makes our lives more enjoyable. We both are experiencing the same uplifting feelings after exercising; like father, like daughter.

Recently my son also informed me about experiencing positive effects from exercising. Since his work is demanding, he struggles with finding the time to exercise. When he can, he feels much better after completing his own routine. Both my children are of mature age where physical exercise is important for maintaining and improving their health. I'm convinced that it also improves their mental health as well.

I now enjoy walking quickly. For many years, I jogged. At this stage of my life, walking is preferred since my right side can cause me discomfort and my knee is not completely healed. My wife is a dedicated walker. She does take long walks and I have accompanied her on many. After injuring her ankle, she was not able to return to the fitness center until only recently. After completing an exercise class, she told me how good it felt. She can now combine her love of walking and yoga with other exercises.

I am happy knowing that my family is engaged in doing things that improve their lives and overall health. Their desire to be fit can influence others they know to do the same. There is much in life about what we do that has some impact on others.

33

$\mathcal{B}$enefits from Exercising

As indicated earlier, there are many benefits associated with becoming fit. I feel it leads to more happiness-feeling better, being more mentally alert, and having more energy to enjoy friends and family.

As I reflect on the physical and psychological setbacks I have experienced during my life, I realize that being in good physical condition helped me recover faster. After the most recent injury, I often thought about when I could actually return to the gym. When I finally did return, I had to start slowly and not rush into it. As I made progress I began to feel both gratification and relief; every step forward was exciting. In all aspects of our lives we are challenged to find the energy to overcome obstacles. Finding the resolve to face one challenge seems to increase the resolve to tackle others.

Those who have lived with injury or illness and through exercise managed to achieve a healthy life have much to offer. By being available to others who may require encouragement, we often become aware of our own struggles, defeats and victories. Assisting others to discover their inner strengths and resolve becomes a reward for our own journey. When I can help others, I find myself renewed and even able to discover my inner strengths. In addition, assisting others to discover their inner strength and resolve to move out of despair is our reward for being there for them. We may find a renewed self within us. Being able to conquer our fears and discover our inner strengths can be a game changer.

As I wrote earlier about my wife suffering a broken ankle and me experiencing a split ligament across my right knee, we rewarded our recoveries with a trip to the Galapagos Islands in the spring of 2017. We were able to participate in the voyage to many islands and it was a wonderful experience to climb to the tops of volcanoes and also swim with turtles, sea lions and millions of fish. We feel blessed to have had such an active and beautiful adventure.

34

$\mathcal{W}$ho I Am - can we ever know?

$\mathbf{W}$riting this book where I focus on exercising has been a journey of introspection. Ultimately, I have come to know myself better. I also want to add that I would not have come this far in life without a spiritual life. This period has tested me in important ways, especially being thankful for my recovery and the resolve to regain fitness. I feel injuries can help us to gain insight to who we are and allow us to identify inner strengths we were not aware we possessed. My desire to regain being fit eventually triumphed over feelings of despair and also led to a better understanding of who I am. I have been able to achieve much success and can relish in this road back. Being aware of the mystery of life also enabled me to realize that I cannot control every setback.

This brings the book to an end. I feel all who read this personal history about exercising following injuries will discover similar pathways to being healthy and fit. In addition, I attempted to share about obstacles in my life that I'm challenged to overcome. Even though I have reached specific goals, there are others that include being able to listen to the desires of others who seek to realize their dream to be fit and healthy.

To my readers, I wish you much success and hope I may meet you in a fitness center, swimming pool, on a forest trail, or attempting to catch the elusive fish. Good Luck!

This is a photo of me in 2016.

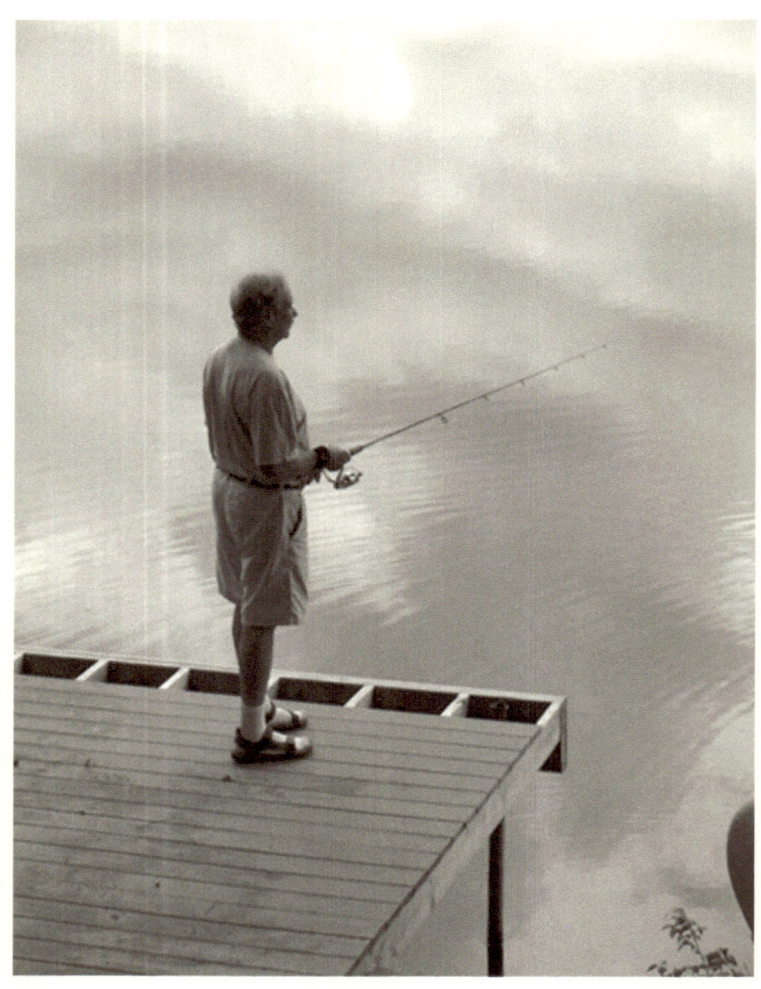

Fini

About the Author

D r. Robert Beauchamp has extensive experience in the fields of geology, environmental science, and education. He was employed as a geologist and oceanographer with the US government. His travels and efforts brought him face-to-face with environmental issues. He went on to become a professor and director of the Environmental Management program at the University of Maryland University College. He developed a team of adjunct faculty who brought real-world environmental experience and background to the classroom. His faculty assisted him to accomplish the program's overreaching goal, which was to continually respond to current environmental issues and future challenges by developing new courses, including adding pertinent topics in existing courses. He continues to teach part-time.

Dr. Beauchamp published a significant number of papers on environmental issues and technologies in peer-reviewed journals. At invitation, he also presented the results of his research on new and emerging environmental technologies at professional conferences. He currently resides in the Washington, DC, area.

www.ingramcontent.com/pod-product-compliance
Lightning Source LLC
Chambersburg PA
CBHW050400290526
45786CB00003B/1067